JOY

The story of a dolphin trainer,
filmmaker, and cancer survivor.

JOY CLAUSEN SOTO

ISBN: 978-1-7362523-0-7

Joy Clausen Soto
San Diego, California

The author is grateful for permission to quote lyrics from the following songs:

Bless The Broken Road
Words and Music by Marcus Hummon, Bobby Boyd and Jeff Hanna Copyright ©
1994 by Universal Music - Careers, Floyd's Dream Music and Jeff Diggs Music All
Rights for Floyd's Dream Music Administered by Universal Music - Careers All
Rights for Jeff Diggs Music Administered by BMG Rights Management (US) LLC
International Copyright Secured All Rights Reserved
Reprinted by Permission of Hal Leonard LLC

Come Pick Me Up
Words and Music by Ryan Adams and Van Alston Copyright © 2000 Barland Music
and Boxorice Music All Rights Administered by BMG Rights Management (US)
LLC All Rights Reserved Used by Permission
Reprinted by Permission of Hal Leonard LLC

Borderline
Words and Music by Reggie Lucas Copyright © 1984 by Universal Music - Careers
International Copyright Secured All Rights Reserved
Reprinted by Permission of Hal Leonard LLC

I Can See Clearly Now
Words and Music by JOHNNY NASH
Copyright © 1972 (Renewed) NASHCO MUSIC
All Rights for the World Outside of North America
Administered by WARNER/CHAPPELL MUSIC, INC.
All Rights Reserved
Used By Permission of ALFRED MUSIC

*To all of the people who undertook
a mission to save my life, thank you.
From the bottom of my heart and
the depths of my soul, thank you.*

TABLE OF CONTENTS

PHOTOGRAPHS

JOY

CHAPTER ONE

Eight Seconds

"Are you okay, Joy?" Kevin turned to ask while driving. The streetlights made his hair glow red.

"Yup," I responded as I curled up in the back seat of his Camaro with my seatbelt on.

"Don't worry. We're almost there. Kevin is pretty much driving like a bat out of hell," Brian assured me as he tightly gripped the handle above the passenger side door. It was the fastest that Kevin had driven with me in the car. What normally took over an hour to drive during the day only took thirty minutes at 1 in the morning.

When we arrived at Children's Hospital Los Angeles, Kevin dropped us off at the main entrance where we usually entered, while he parked the car. The hospital was empty. Lights were off in the areas where there were normally employees checking people in during the day.

As we made our way down the hallway, my legs started to buckle over and over again. I was too weak to walk. Brian and I looked at each other helplessly, then at the long hallway in front of us. No one was around to help, and he had my overnight bag in one hand and a pillow in the other. Then Brian started to rearrange things. He threw my bag over his shoulder and shoved the pillow under his arm.

"Alright, here we go," he said as he wrapped his free arm around my waist.

He helped me walk the entire way to the emergency room. I thought back to when Brian walked me back to my dorm one night in college to make sure I was safe. That was back when I was healthy and had long, curly brown hair and a ton of energy. I never expected my life to take a turn like this.

"Next," the lady behind the counter said. "Hi, I'm being treated here for cancer, and I'm supposed to come in tomorrow for a blood transfusion, but I got a fever."

That's all I had to say, "fever." It's one of the first things that you hear from doctors and nurses. "Now, if you get a fever at some point, go straight to the hospital." A fever is a big deal when you have cancer. Chemotherapy knocks down your blood counts, which means that your body's white blood cells that normally attack intruders aren't there in high enough numbers to help you. A simple fever could kill you.

"Can I lie down out there while we're waiting?" I asked the lady who was checking me in. I pointed to a wooden bench outside of the ER.

"Out there?" she asked.

"Yeah, I'm just really weak, and I'd rather lie down while we're waiting," I said as I put my hand on my throat and winced in pain. She looked out into the hallway at the bench and reluctantly agreed.

"Yeah, okay. I'll let them know you're out there," she said.

"Thank you."

I turned to walk toward the bench, but my knees gave out again, and I started to fall. Suddenly I felt an arm wrap around my back.

"I've got you," Brian said with a smile.

He helped me walk the rest of the way to the bench.

It was my first ER visit. To be honest, I was scared, but I came prepared for a stay. I had my pillow, favorite blanket, a bag full of clothes (mainly pajamas - it wasn't the Oscars), and my trusty medical notebook filled with copies of all of my medical information.

I placed my pillow on the bench, then did a sort of tuck and roll to lie down, pulled my favorite blanket up, and voila, a makeshift bed.

Kevin walked up right after I nuzzled into my bench/bed.

"They put her out here? Are you kidding me?" he asked Brian in disbelief.

"I asked to be out here. I wanted to lie down," I said in a weak, shaky voice.

Brian and Kevin stood there waiting for a doctor to come out while I took up the only available seating with my new bed. It was getting more and more painful to talk because I had mucositis, an inflammation of the mouth, throat, and basically the entire GI track due to chemotherapy. Think of the feeling you have when you get strep throat, and you will have some idea of what it feels like to have mucositis.

I waved my hand to signal to the guys that I wanted their attention. They looked at me waving my hand. Next, I decided to use my mean charade skills to let them know what I wanted. I made the sign for movie and then pointed to myself.

They looked at each other, profoundly confused.

"Do you know what she wants?" Brian asked Kevin.

"Umm, I'm not sure," Kevin said slowly while thinking. Then I more emphatically reenacted my on-point charade routine.

"Oh. I think she wants us to videotape her," Brian sighed.

"Is that what you want?" Kevin asked in a bit of disbelief. I nodded my head.

I met Kevin at film school. When I saw his reel I was amazed at what he had directed and I thought he was one of the best filmmakers at school. He reluctantly got out my old Sony camcorder and filmed me for an entire eight seconds. It was probably the saddest I had seen either of them during this whole ordeal. I wasn't thinking that it was too much for them to film this moment.

At twenty-five I was making a documentary on my battle with cancer. I hoped that it would be my very own "Rocky" story, a story of survival. But I knew that there was a chance I might not make it, and so did everyone around me. That's why Kevin only filmed for eight seconds.

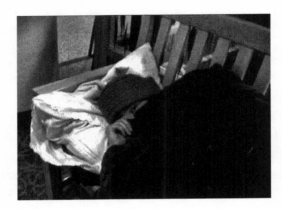

CHAPTER TWO

Two Years Earlier

The pool was half the distance that I needed to swim. I had to hold my breath for at least two lengths of the pool in order to pass the test. Focus, breathe, go for it. I dove in and attempted to hold my breath, but as I pulled my body through the water, I started to crave oxygen. I wanted to keep going, but the urge to breathe was overwhelming.

"Pull, kick, glide... pull, kick, glide." That was what my swim teacher told me to think about during my breaststroke. *Pull, kick, glide...* I kept repeating the words in my mind. "Puhhhhh!" I surfaced and took a deep breath. I swam half the length... half the length? That meant I would not only fail my swim test, but fail miserably. I pulled my body out of the pool, dove back in, and tried to make it further than my first attempt. Other people were in the pool playing and swimming. They had no idea that I was preparing for a job interview. This would be the most important day at the pool that I would ever have in my life.

Practice was over. It was time to go to the airport and catch a stand-by flight. I sat at the airport and watched full flight after full flight leave without me to San Diego.

"How's it going?" my boyfriend, Jerry, asked me over the phone.

"Well, I'm still in Chicago, so not great. I think I'm just going to come home, and we can rent a movie."

"Are there any more flights left?"

"Yeah, there is one more, but it's not until 10:50 tonight, and it's a packed flight too."

"Stay, and try to get on that one. You're already there. You might as well stay for one more flight. We can watch a movie another night," he said to me.

He was right. Of course he was right, but part of me started to think that maybe this wasn't meant to be. I mean I couldn't even hold my breath for one length of a small pool much less 120 feet underwater. Why was I even getting on that plane?

The 10:50 p.m. flight had openings. I was on my way to San Diego. Now there was that small matter of not physically being able to pass the test. I remembered reading that professional basketball players visualize the ball going into the hoop before actually shooting the ball. Visualization is a technique that a lot of athletes use. So I tried that. I sat on the plane and visualized myself swimming underwater, wanting to give up, but continuing on and not giving into the urge to breathe. I practiced holding my breath while timing myself on my oversized, silver Casio watch. I visualized diving to the bottom of the pool and imagined what it would feel like to dive that deep, expecting for my ears to bother me, but pushing through it to get to the bottom. It's all I did the entire flight. I visualized over and over again. Holding my breath again and again. Taking the test again and again in my mind.

"Is this a vacation for you?" a man across the aisle asked.

"Oh, no. I'm going for a job interview," I replied.

"Well, good luck. What's the job?" he asked.

"A dolphin trainer position at SeaWorld," I said with a big smile.

"Oh, that sounds like a dream job," he said.

"I know, but they need me to take a swim test. If I pass the test, I think I have a good chance of getting the job because I used to work with dolphins in Hawaii. The only problem is I tried passing the test this morning, and I couldn't do it. I didn't even come close. So right now I am practicing by holding my breath and imagining myself taking the test in my mind," I blurted out to him.

"I was a Navy Seal, and we would use visualization techniques," he said.

"Oh really?" I said. Apparently, I was onto something.

"Yeah, yeah, and holding your breath will help you improve your lung capacity."

"Oh, great."

"Well, I'll leave you to it. Good luck," he said.

I went back to holding my breath and timing myself.

If I could just pass this swim test, I had a good shot of getting a position there. I had prior experience training dolphins and Hawaiian monk seals in Hawaii. My bachelor's degree was in psychology from Chaminade University. Psychology is the most useful degree to have because positive reinforcement is the foundation of animal training. Plus, I was getting my master's degree from the University of Chicago in the social sciences. I had a lot of good things going for me. I just had to pull out a miracle and hope that all of this visualization would actually pay off and make up for what I could not do physically.

CHAPTER THREE

The Swim Test

The sound of the wheels screeching as they touched down in San Diego brought me back to the realization that I was actually doing this. I had arrived in San Diego to interview for a job as a SeaWorld trainer. As we were deplaning, I kept holding my breath and timing myself as I waited with my fellow passengers to get off of the plane. I finally made it to my hotel in San Diego around 11:50 p.m. The next morning I got up early and was ready to go to SeaWorld for my 9 a.m. swim test. I grabbed a taxi, carrying my suitcase with me so I could catch a flight back to Chicago right after the test.

In Human Resources I sat with about a dozen other applicants. "I am so nervous." I heard one applicant say. I was too, but I didn't want to feed into that energy. I just kept myself busy with some work for my master's degree. I had a book open and read the same paragraph about a dozen times, but of course I wasn't really reading that paragraph. I was still visualizing. With my head down in the book in front of me I looked un-approachable. That was good. I didn't want to admit that I was nervous. I had to keep in the zone, and that is exactly what I did.

"Okay, everyone, thank you for being here. Please grab your belongings and follow us." It was early in the morning before SeaWorld opened. We walked through the empty park until we reached Dolphin Stadium. I remember certain images: wet pavement, sand, a lighthouse, the trainer's locker room, and of course the main show pool. We changed in the locker rooms. I wore a one-piece bathing suit that my mom had given me. It was bright yellow, pink, and orange all swirled together. One trainer walked in to grab something from her blue locker. "Good luck!" she said as she walked by us in her SeaWorld wetsuit.

We met in front of the locker rooms, clad in our bathing suits. Then they led us over a bridge to the main show pool. There were dolphins and pilot whales in the adjoining pools that we passed, clicking and whistling as we walked by. We all gathered by the show pool.

"Alright, you are going to take the test in groups of two. For the first part of the test you will be swimming freestyle to the acrylic (the glass-like area) and back to stage in under one minute and twenty seconds. Next, will be the underwater breath hold, once again, swimming to the acrylic and back. Now, don't get to the acrylic and take a breath. The test is for you to hold your breath there and back. Finally, after both of those parts are completed, we will have you swim to the middle of the pool and dive down to the bottom. You need to touch the bottom to pass this part of the test. We'll have someone watching from the acrylic to make sure you touch the bottom. Any questions?" the trainer asked.

No one had any questions. "Alright, you two will be in the first group." She pointed to two people and then went on pairing everyone. I was in the last group, which was good. I got to see how people performed on the test.

We all passed the freestyle swim with flying colors. Next was the underwater breath hold. The first few groups of girls passed like it was nothing. As the test went on, some of the girls came up early for air. The group ahead of us started. "You can get in the water now," the trainer instructed us. We got in and held onto the stage while waiting for the girls ahead of us to finish their swim. I could feel the adrenaline pumping through my body. The girls were almost done. One girl came up for air early. The other finished. The trainer closest to us yelled, "Go!" I took a deep breath, sank down in the water, and pushed with all of my might off of the wall with both feet.

Borderline, feels like I'm going to lose my mind. You just keep on pushing my love over the borderline. The lyrics from Madonna's song kept repeating in my head. I sang to myself to keep my mind off of that all-important thing required for living, oxygen. I could hear the sound of clicks and whistles from the dolphins and whales as I swam. I wanted to come up for air, but I wanted the job more. A little bit of suffering was worth it. *You just keep on pushing my love... over the borderline.* I reached the acrylic! That was already twice as far as I had gone the day before, but I wasn't done... I still had to swim that same length back to stage without coming up for air. I turned underwater and pushed off of the acrylic. *You just keep on pushing my love...* I pulled and kicked faster and faster.

Come up for air. It will be so nice to breathe again, my body told me.

Never! I am not coming up until I touch that stage! my mind yelled back.

The swim back to stage felt so long. In my mind/body battle, I somehow got off course and veered toward the pool where the animals were. Luckily, a trainer splashed her hand in the water to help redirect me. I readjusted my course. I could see the stage. I was almost there. I reached out my hand and kicked hard until I felt the wall, then came up for air. I did it! I passed the underwater swim! Little did anyone know that this had been physically impossible for me just twenty-four hours earlier. I pulled my body out of the water and waited for the next part of the test.

The final part was the twenty-six foot dive down to the bottom. My ears normally started to hurt at six feet in a regular pool. I had never been more than twenty feet underwater, and that was on SCUBA in the ocean.

More people were not passing this part of the test. They would come up with pain in their ears and then swim back to stage. "Come on out," a trainer called to me from the middle of the pool. I swam out to her. "Whenever you're ready," she told me as we both sculled over the deepest part of the pool. I took a few breaths, then one final breath and dove down.

As I pulled my body through the water, all I could think was, *Oh My Goodness, this is a lot of water to get through. Pull, kick, pull, kick.* My ears started to hurt. I tried swallowing to equalize, which was my normal way of equalizing when scuba diving, but it didn't work. This was my one shot at passing the test and working at SeaWorld. I couldn't give up. I kept pulling myself down, deeper, and deeper. Then I heard a stream of pops from my ear. Pop-pop-pop-pop-pop-pop-pop-pop-pop. That can't be good, but I wasn't going to stop. Almost there... just a few more strokes. I pulled with all of my might, and then I was there. I touched the grate at the bottom of the pool and looked around in amazement that I had actually done it. I made it to the bottom! Then I turned and got as close to the grate as I could to get a good push off the bottom. That's when I looked UP for the first time.

Now, if there is ever a time to be calm and not freak out, this would be one of those times. There was twenty-six feet of water above me. I wanted air, but coming up early wasn't a choice I had in this situation. I went into a calm state as I kicked up to the surface. Then about half way up, I felt my buoyancy kick in. My body was being pulled to the surface as I helped it along with kicks. I could see the sky through the water get clearer and clearer, I was almost there. "Puhhh!" I gasped for air as I came up from my journey to another world. "Great job! You can swim in now," the trainer told me after I surfaced.

After the swim test we went back to the locker rooms. Some girls were crying. "I'm so mad at myself. I trained for eight months," one girl said. I felt sorry for her, but I also felt proud of myself for doing the impossible and passing the test. I put myself out there and went for it, even though the odds of succeeding were extremely low.

We walked out of the locker rooms and waited to hear the results. "You all did a great job out there. Here are the applicants who will be moving on to the interview portion." I waited, listening to names get called that I didn't recognize. Then I heard, "Joy Clausen." I had done it! I passed the SeaWorld swim test and made it to the interview process!

I called my dad and stepmom to let them know what happened. They were so excited for me.

"You did it! You really did it, you little rascal!" my dad said while chuckling in disbelief.

"Yeah, I can't believe it! Now I have to get ready for the interview," I said.

"Okay, well, my best advice for you during any interview is to just be yourself. Let them see your personality."

"Okay, I'll try. Thank you, Dad. I love you."

"I love you too, sweetheart. Good luck!"

Then my stepmom who has been in my life since I was three years old got on the line.

"You did it, you little devil, you!" she said. "Okay, but now you have the interview. They are looking for a SeaWorld trainer, so be their perfect SeaWorld trainer," she said.

"Okay," I responded.

"Hey, I am so proud of you. Good luck!" she told me before getting off the phone.

The interview seemed to go well. After each answer the curator and trainer would smile and look at each other. The interview ended, and I felt like I had done as well as I could have.

After the interview Allison from HR walked me out to the front of SeaWorld to show me where to catch a taxi.

"So, do you want to know how you did?" she asked after a brief moment of silence.

"Sure..." I replied.

"It was the best interview we have had. Your answers were perfect," she said.

I got in a taxi and went straight to the airport smiling from ear to ear.

"I did it! I passed the swim test!" I said to Jerry from a payphone in the airport. "I'm catching a flight back to Chicago right now. I am so excited!"

"That is so great, Hon. Aren't you happy you waited for that last flight now?" he said.

"Yes! Yes, I am! Thank you!"

The days went by, and of course I started to think that maybe I didn't get the job. With each day that passed my excitement level dropped, and doubt crept into my mind. *Who was I kidding, me, a SeaWorld trainer? Well, at least I tried,* I thought. I was still proud of myself for trying and somehow miraculously passing the swim test, but that interview did go well, so well that one of the people in the interview felt compelled to tell me. *Will they call me to let me know if I didn't get it?* I wondered. On the eleventh day of my downward spiral:

"Hi, I'm calling for Joy Clausen," someone said on the phone.

"Yes, this is she," I responded.

"Hi, this is Allison from SeaWorld, I am calling to offer you a full-time position as an associate trainer at the Dolphin Interaction Program here in San Diego. If you need time to think about it..."

"Yes! Yes, I will take the position! Thank you so much!" I said.

I called Jerry at work, "They offered me the position! They want me to be a trainer in San Diego," I said.

"Wow, that's great. Wow. Okay, let's take the weekend to think about it," he said.

"Okay," I responded even though I had already accepted the position. It's just that this was SeaWorld! This was my dream job, and as much as I loved Jerry, I needed to find a job that I loved. If I couldn't find something that fulfilled me, then I couldn't be happy. We got together with his family and discussed things over dinner.

"Well, this is a once in a lifetime opportunity," his stepmom said as we all talked together.

"I know," I said.

"So, would you have a long distance relationship?" his father asked us.

"Well, we will have to figure that out," Jerry said. We both knew long distance relationships didn't work. If I took the job, that would be the end of us.

Later in the car Jerry said, "I think you should take it. It's your dream job. You've always dreamed of working for SeaWorld." I quietly nodded with tears in my eyes. It was the beginning of the end, but that is the beautiful thing when you care for someone, you want them to be happy above all else. We were good friends for a very long time before we started dating, so we could go back to being good friends again.

I moved to San Diego to start my new job and my new life.

CHAPTER FOUR

A Dream Come True

"What size wetsuit do you wear?" a trainer named Kym asked.
"Oh, I'm not sure," I replied.

"Hmmm, okay, let's try a five and see how that fits," she said.

I was in the Dolphin Stadium trainers' locker room at SeaWorld San Diego. I was in the trainers' locker room because it was my first day as a SEAWORLD TRAINER!

I pulled and tugged and contorted my way into the size 5 wetsuit. A couple of times I lost my grip and you could hear a loud snap come from the bathroom where I was changing. Then, I finally got into the wetsuit and walked out to show Kym.

"Hmm, I think you can go a size smaller. Let me get you a 3 to try on," she said, as she looked me up and down, analyzing the fit of my wetsuit.

Smaller? Oh no, no, I don't want to get out of this wetsuit. It took me forever to get into it. I finally feel like a real SeaWorld trainer, and I have no idea how I'm going to get this thing off, I frantically thought.

"You know what? I really like the way this one fits," I said to her.

"Oh, okay. Great," she said. She found some wetsuit booties for me to wear on my feet, and I was off to walk outside the locker room as a real SeaWorld trainer for the first time.

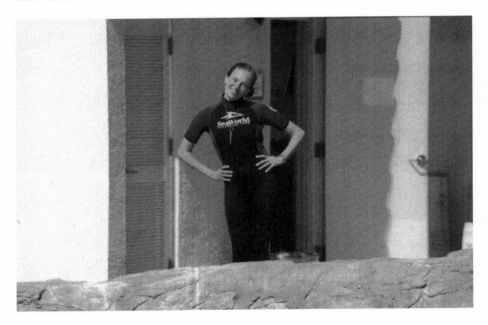

On my first day I went to orientation with Christine, a tall, blonde who was hired to work at Dolphin Show. As we walked to orientation, she leaned in as if she were telling me a secret, "Did you know that we were the only two trainers in the entire company to get hired as full-time associates? Everyone else came in as seasonal apprentices." Her eyes were wide with excitement, and a look of, "Oh, heck yea!" I instantly liked her.

"Are you serious?" I asked.

"Yup, out of the entire company," she said, as she made a circle with her finger to encompass all three SeaWorlds.

It was so easy to make friends at SeaWorld. Everyone was so nice and welcoming. We were all bonded by our love for animals and our unique jobs. I became good friends with everyone I worked with.

One day as we were about to start a session with the dolphins, my supervisor, Bob, turned to me and said, "Why don't you footpush her into the next pool?"

"Footpush her?" I asked. A footpush is when the dolphin pushes your foot with the tip of its mouth. It... is... awesome. I'd seen people do footpushes, but that was it. "I've never done one before," I said to him.

"Okay! I'll show you what it looks like," he said, and with that he did a perfect dive into the water next to the dolphin he had in front of him and stuck out his foot. The dolphin came up behind him and pushed on his foot. He did a surface dive, and suddenly he was flying underwater with a dolphin pushing him from behind. The next thing I knew he had surfaced in the adjacent pool and was footpushing around the pool. All I could see was white water and Bob flying around. Then he swam to the side of the pool and fed her some fish. It looked incredible.

Bob got out of the water and ran back to me. "Okay, you want to give it a try?" he asked, out of breath from what he had just done.

"Sure," I said with a combined feeling of excitement and fright.

"Just jump in, stick out your foot, and then duck your head down and steer her to the other pool," he said.

"Okay." I jumped in and stuck out my foot. She started pushing me toward the opening for the next pool, but then I bent my knee and broke off.

"What happened?" he asked, his head cocked to the side with a look of bewilderment.

"I think I need to back up a little and try it," I said, but it was also because I was a little scared. I got out of the water, walked down a little further, and then jumped in. I stuck out my foot, and suddenly I was flying. I ducked my head under water and saw the opening for the other pool. I directed my body toward the opening, and before I knew it I was in the next pool. "Mewwwwww!" I could hear the dolphin squeal with excitement as we glided through the water. We surfaced together and she was still squealing. It was the same excitement I had in my heart. I had the biggest smile humanly possible. It was absolutely incredible. This was my job. They were paying me to do this. I was so happy.

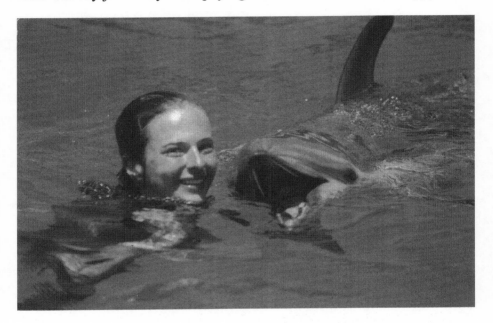

CHAPTER FIVE

Itchy Soul

My dad gave me my first video camera when I was in college. It was an old Sony camcorder that he had owned and passed on to me. I didn't use it much at first, but then I started videotaping my adventures with marine mammals. Eventually, I figured out how to edit without using a computer. I would hook up my video camera to the VCR and stereo (for music) and edit the video into something fun for my dad to watch. Eventually, I made a film for my co-workers at SeaWorld.

"Quiet, everyone! The video is starting," Kym said to everyone at the party. "Mike, can you turn off the lights?" With that the lights went out, and the whole room of about twenty trainers fixated on a screen showing the movie that I had put together.

Then magic happened. They started to laugh. Any talking that had been going on before died down, and they were transfixed by my video. I looked around and saw the beautiful silhouettes of people turned toward the light of the television screen, all laughing and reacting in unison.

"Joy, you did this?" Jim turned to me and asked.

"Yeah," I replied.

"Wow, this is incredible," he said.

"That's my Joyee!" Christine said as she put her arm around me in a prideful hug. The best part was when it ended and they rewound it and played it again... and again. Wow, what an incredible feeling to create something and to get that kind of a response!

I worked at SeaWorld for a couple of years, but found myself daydreaming about how I would edit videos when I got home. This is when I started to get an itchy soul, a feeling of restlessness. I was happy at SeaWorld, but I didn't know if this was what I was meant to do for the rest of my life, especially when all I could think about was editing films.

I kept making videos in my free time, including one for my mom's side of the family. It showed everyone from my grandmother and grandfather to my younger brother and sister. I showed it to my aunt and uncle, and my aunt's best friend Genya (my mom wasn't there because she lived in Hawaii). By the end of the video I looked around and what I can only describe as a look of shock was on everyone's face. This wasn't a typical response to one of my films, hmmm. I wasn't quite sure how to take it. Later on I found out that my aunt and uncle had seen footage of their parents that they had never seen before. They were blown away by the video. Genya grabbed my hands and looked into my eyes.

"This is what you should be doing," she said.

"Joy, that was unbelievable. Have you thought about going to film school?" my aunt asked.

"I've thought about doing more with video," I said.

"This is a talent, Joy. You have a talent," Genya said as she held my hands and looked into my eyes.

"Did you know there is a film school just up the road in Santa Barbara?" Aunt Susan said with a smile.

"Oh, there is? No, I didn't know that."

"You could go to school in Santa Barbara and live here with me in Ventura, rent-free, and I can help you with tuition," she said as she worked out all of the details in real time. My aunt had short jet-black hair, a light complexion, light brown eyes, and ruby red lips. She was an amazing person who worked her way up and became a vice president at MCA Recreation Services (the company that owned Universal Studios). She was tough, kind, and the type of person that made things happen.

I went back to work and thought about her offer. I loved my friends, I loved the animals, I loved my job, but all I could think about was film-making. My aunt had offered for me to stay with her rent-free and to pay for film school. I didn't have a road map in life telling me what to do, but I did have a path unfolding before me that I could not ignore.

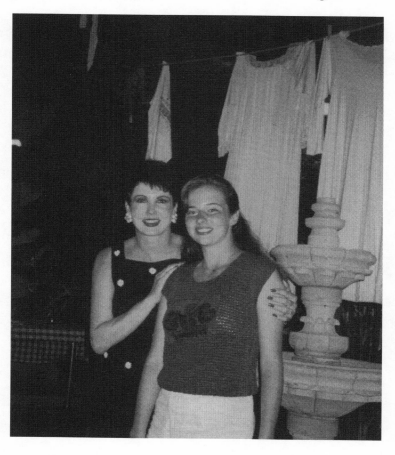

CHAPTER SIX

The Last Day

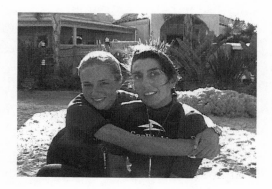

"A dream is a wish from the heart, so always follow your dreams," my friend Ann said as I hugged her on my last day at SeaWorld while another trainer, Mike, videotaped us. Ann was quirky and wonderful.

I met Ann at a SeaWorld softball game. She was sitting in the stands watching her fiancé play.

"You work at the Dolphin Interaction Program, right?" she asked me.

"Yes, I do," I said.

"Do you love it?" she asked with a smile and wonderment in her eyes.

"Yes! The dolphins are incredible, and the people are too. I really love it," I said.

"That's what I thought. It's my dream to work there one day. I told them in my review that I want to go to the Dolphin Interaction Program. Maybe one day I'll be working with you," she said with a big smile.

"That would be great. I hope you get to come to our area," I said.

Ann did come to our area and she became one of my favorite people to work with. She was humble and eager to become a better trainer. When she got notes after a training session (and we ALL got notes after a training session), she would write down what she learned in a notebook in order to get better. The final thing about Ann, she was quirky.

When Ann first got to our area she was about to get married, so we got to hear about every aspect and I mean EVERY aspect of her wedding dress. We would get out of the water from a training session, listen to our notes from other trainers, and then when there was a moment of silence she would change the subject to her wedding dress. "Have I told you about the lace?" she would ask. "Oh, and the gloves. The gloves go to about here... " I would hear her say to someone as I walked away to wash buckets. "Did I tell you that I have two trains? The second one is entirely translucent and trails two feet further behind the first train, making the statement, 'you thought the dress was spectacular... look at ME!'" It was pretty much that scene from Forest Gump, but instead of shrimp it was her wedding dress. She was very excited about getting married and over the moon about her wedding dress.

I think that is what I loved the most about my co-workers, they all had these wonderful personalities. Life was good with my friends at SeaWorld. I was walking away from a gold mine.

"I'm going to be leaving, so I don't get to see you anymore. I'm going to miss you so much," I whispered to my favorite dolphin, Bullet, as I hugged her with tears in my eyes. I pulled my face away to look at her.

"You know you're amazing, don't you?" I whispered to her as I noticed my tearful reflection on her slick skin.

Then I said goodbye to another one of my favorite animals, a small common dolphin named Buster. Buster was tiny compared to the other animals. He had stripes down his side and weighed a fraction of what the bottlenose dolphins weighed. I lined him up in front of me and gave him a big hug, lifting him out of the water a bit. I could feel his heart beating between his pectoral flippers. Every time I kissed him, he would make a raspberry vocalization and Mike, who was videotaping this moment, decided to say "Goodbye" in a funny, deep voice every time Buster made this sound, which was a lot. "Goodbye. Goodbye. Goodbye," Mike said over and over again, matching Buster's vocalizations. It started to make me laugh through my tears. It's amazing how a friend can do that, how they can lighten the mood to ease your soul. "Buster, I'm going to miss you. I hope I'm making the right decision. If only you could talk, Buster," I said to him as I laughed through my tears. Then I gave him one final point away to another trainer and got out of the water for the last time. I ended my last day as a SeaWorld trainer hoping that I was choosing the right path in life.

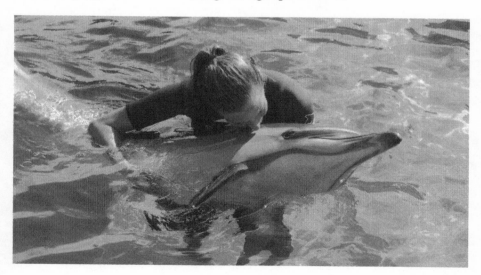

CHAPTER SEVEN

Film School

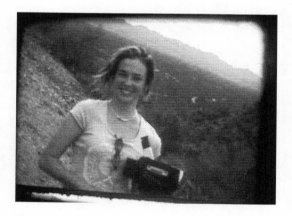

I was about to turn twenty-five and embarking on a big change in life. Film school started, and I found myself in class with people who were younger than me. I had never been the oldest one. In fact, I had always been the youngest one in school, even among my co-workers at SeaWorld.

I sat down in my first class and waited for our teacher, Mr. Schwartz, to show up.

"So, where are you from?" a guy sitting next to me asked.

"San Diego. How about you?" I asked.

"Orange County. Did you go to UCSD? I have some friends that go there," he said.

"No."

"So, what were you doing down there?"

"I was a dolphin trainer at SeaWorld."

"What? You were a dolphin trainer? Why would you leave a job as a dolphin trainer?" he asked, making it clear that he would not do the same thing.

"Well, to be a filmmaker! To follow another dream," I said, in my majestic, "I am woman and I can do whatever I put my mind to" kind of way.

"Did you get to swim with them?" he asked.

"Uhhuh," I said as I nodded with a smile.

"Now THAT is MY dream job!" he said.

I was so excited to be in film school, but no one else could understand why I would leave a job where I swam with dolphins. A pang of "I hope I didn't make a mistake," went through my body.

While at film school I learned how to use cameras and lighting. They had an equipment checkout area where we could borrow lights, cameras, microphones, and lots of other things for our projects. The checkout guys were always super nice and helpful. I got to know them by name.

"Thanks for showing me how to set up the lighting kit, Ellis," I said. Ellis worked in equipment checkout. He wore glasses, had a shaved head, a thin build, and was slightly taller than I was.

"No problem, anytime. You just..." A tall man with dark brown hair interrupted Ellis.

"Hey, you want to see what I'm working on?" he asked me with a gleam of excitement and a touch of mischief in his eyes. I didn't know him, but he really seemed excited about his project.

"Sure," I said. "Thanks again for everything, Ellis," I said as I started to walk off.

Ellis didn't stay in checkout but followed me and lingered around. I was about to go see what this person was so excited about when Ellis stopped me, then turned his body away from where I was headed and nonchalantly whispered, "Joy, that's John. That guy is a bit of a jerk. Be careful."

John popped his head out of the editing room, "Are you coming?" he asked.

"Yeah," I said. "Okay, thank you for telling me," I said as I turned around and walked towards the editing room to see John's work. I could feel Ellis just standing there helplessly as he watched me walk away.

Later on John asked me out on a date, and before I knew it we were a couple. We took dance lessons together, swam in his pool, and went out on the main strip in Santa Barbara to have drinks. He even picked up groceries and cooked dinner for me. It was nice.

One day at dance lessons I was feeling exhausted. I had been trying to get over a cough and cold. As I looked in the mirror at dance class, I noticed dark circles under my eyes, and every movement just took the wind out of me. "Hey, would you mind if we just went home and rested? I'm really tired," I said.

"Oh, really? Okay, yeah, let's go," he said and took my hand as we walked out of the class. "I'm sorry you're not feeling good."

"It's okay," I said out of breath as I walked down the stairs. I didn't realize how exhausted I was. We went back to his house and watched part of a movie.

"Alright, well... I should go now. I have a long drive tomorrow to see my uncle," I said.

"Awe, so soon?"

"Yeah, I've got to get ready for Thanksgiving. When are you heading out to see your mom?" I asked.

"Tomorrow, I think around 11."

"Okay, well, I'll see you after Thanksgiving!" He walked me to the door. I gave him a hug goodbye. As I turned to leave, he stopped me.

"You make me so happy," he said with a big smile as he looked into my eyes.

"I do?" I asked with a smile.

Then he gave me another big hug and said, "Yes, you really do." He looked so happy. It was a really nice moment, and it made me happy too.

That was the last time we talked before Thanksgiving break.

CHAPTER EIGHT

Thanksgiving

"**O**kay, Joyous, we'll see you at 2 o'clock. Make sure you bring an appetite because Aunt Julie is making us a feast," Uncle David said to me over the phone.

I packed up my green Toyota Tercel with an overnight bag and a roll of toilet paper, so I could blow my nose during the drive. This cough was not going away. In fact, it seemed to be getting worse instead of better.

I jumped into my car and made some phone calls to wish people a happy Thanksgiving. I called Ann. "Hello?" she answered.

"Hi, Ann, it's Joy. I just wanted to wish you a happy Thanksgiving and tell you I am grateful to have you in my life," I said.

"Awww, I'm grateful for you too, Joy. Whatcha doin' for Thanksgiving?"

"I'm going to my uncle's, and you?"

"Oh, we're going to my parent's house later today."

"Okay, well, have fun. I just wanted to tell you how much you mean to me. I'll talk to you later, Ann," I said as I got off the phone with her. It was Thanksgiving, and I wanted to tell people how thankful I was for them.

I decided to stop by the retirement home to see my grandpa. In all honesty I felt a little sick to my stomach going there. I wasn't sure how it would be to see him. The last time I visited him with my aunt he was just staring at the clock on the wall. It seemed like he was watching the minutes pass until he died. He was in his 90's and had already said goodbye to his wife, my grandma, a while back when she passed away. Grandpa Len had been a priest in the Catholic Church, but left the church in order to marry my grandmother. Now he just spent his time waiting to see her again.

"Hi, Grandpa," I said as I slowly walked into his room. "It's me, Joy."

"Oh, Joy! Hi, how have you been?" he said in a shaky voice while trying to sit up in bed.

"I'm good. I just wanted to stop by and wish you a happy Thanksgiving."

"Oh, thank you. Are you having Thanksgiving at Susan's?"

"No, she's out of town. I'm going to Uncle David's house," I said as I turned my head away to cough.

"That sounds nice. Tell me, how are the dolphins in San Diego?" he asked with a big smile.

"Oh, they're great, but I don't work with them anymore. I actually live up here now! I'm going to film school and living with Aunt Susan," I said.

"Do you still get to swim with those dolphins?" he asked, not too interested in what I had just told him.

"No, not anymore."

"Well, I'll bet they miss you."

"Yeah, they probably do," I said with a smile. "Okay, well, I just wanted to wish you a happy Thanksgiving and tell you that I love you. I should get back on the road to Uncle David's house. I love you, Grandpa." I leaned over and gave him a kiss on his unshaven cheek.

He grabbed my hand with his shaky one, "God bless you, sweetheart. Hey, thank you for coming to see me," he said as he held onto my hand and looked into my eyes.

"Of course, I love you, Grandpa," I said. Then I got back on the road to my uncle's house.

"Hello," my mom answered. She was in Hawaii, so we wouldn't be together for Thanksgiving.

"Hi, Mom! I wanted to call and wish you a happy Thanksgiving! I love you!" I said.

"Oh, sweetie, I love you too. Thank you so much for calling me."

"So, what are you doing for Thanksgiving?" I asked.

"Oh, I don't have any big plans. I might go over to Chandra's house later on today. What about you?" she asked.

"I'm going to Uncle David's house," I said.

"Oh, that sounds nice," she said, and with that the conversation stalled.

"Okay, well, I love you, Mom. Have a great day," I said to her as I got off the phone. My mom never seemed to have much to say over the phone to me. I asked her why this was when I first noticed it in college. She said it was because she was "phone-a-phobic" a fear of phones. I'm not making this up (although, I am fairly certain that word is made up).

My parents divorced when I was three, and since then I have always felt like I was the one taking care of her. I remember at three years old being on a small Cessna plane with her at night as we flew out of Massachusetts, away from my dad and into Connecticut. *Now that it's just the two of us, I need to make sure that we're safe*, I thought as I studied her beautiful face.

As a three year old, with feety pajamas on, I would walk around to all of the doors in our house and make sure they were locked to keep us safe. I loved her with all of my heart, but I also worried about her as if I were her mother.

I arrived at my uncle's house.

"Joyous!" Uncle David said as he opened the door and greeted me.

"Hi, Uncle David! Sorry, I'm a little sick," I said to him as I coughed.

"Welcome! We have a big feast so I hope you're hungry," Julie said.

"Oh, I am," I said, and then I started to cough again. As I coughed, I did something I hadn't done before, I put my hand on my throat, right by my clavicle, and to my surprise a lump met my hand. I could feel the blood drain from my face. "I'll be right back," I said as I walked briskly to the bathroom to look at what I just felt. It was a lump under my skin about the size of an egg. It wasn't red, and it didn't hurt when I touched it, but it was hard.

"Did I have this when I walked in?" I asked as I emerged from the bathroom pointing to my new discovery.

"What?" asked Aunt Julie as she got closer.

"This," I said as I pointed to my neck where the lump was.

"No, I don't remember seeing that when you came in." She reached out and touched it.

"I don't know, maybe a spider bite?" she said.

I looked at my uncle. "Did you see this when I came in, Uncle David? Did you notice it?" I asked in an interrogation style.

"No, no, I didn't notice anything," he said.

I sat down on the couch palpating my lump. "It's pretty big. Don't you think you would have noticed it when I walked in?" I asked, unsure of how long it had been there. We sat there for a bit unable to move on to other topics. The lump had taken over.

"You know what? There is an Urgent Care right around the corner. Why don't I take you there, and they can take a look at it," Uncle David suggested.

"Okay, do you think we need to go there?" I asked.

"Well, it doesn't hurt to have someone look at it, and it's five minutes away," he said. We said, "Goodbye," to Julie, who stayed home to finish cooking.

The waiting room at Urgent Care was empty. I picked up a magazine and opened it to a page about leukemia. After reading a few paragraphs, "Joy…" the nurse called. I put down the magazine and followed the nurse to the doctor's exam room while my uncle stayed back in the waiting room.

"I understand you found a lump," the doctor said as he looked at the notes from the nurse.

"Yes, right here on my neck. I coughed and when I put my hand on my throat, which I don't normally do, I felt it. We were thinking maybe it's a spider bite or something?"

The doctor walked over and looked at the lump, then pressed his finger against it. "Does this hurt?" he asked.

"No," I said as I looked straight ahead.

"What about this?" he asked as he pushed his thumb against it with more pressure.

"No," I answered. I have always thought of myself as being healthy and strong. This was just another testament to that fact.

He continued to palpate the lump. "Now does it hurt?" he asked.

"No," I said with increasing pride in my voice. I was feeling pretty tough since it didn't hurt. *Go ahead. Push harder. It doesn't hurt. That's right, I'm strong. He must be impressed,* I thought.

He was quiet as he continued examining my neck. Then he stopped and walked away. I said, "It's good if it doesn't hurt, right?" He was writing down some notes and didn't look at me.

"No, it's not always good if it doesn't hurt."

My stomach dropped. "It's not?" I asked him.

"No, it's not," he said in a serious tone without looking up from his paper, "I'm going to need you to see a doctor on Monday. A doctor that you will be seeing regularly."

My mind jumped to the article I had just read, although I thought I was overreacting. "Do you think it could be leukemia?" I asked. He didn't answer. Instead there was just silence.

Finally he said, "I understand you came with your uncle?"

"Yeah," I said, feeling the tone of our meeting completely change.

"I'd like to speak with him if it is okay with you."

"Yeah, sure." I opened the door that led to the waiting room and saw my uncle look up with a smile. "The doctor wants to speak to you," I said without my usual smile, then walked across the room and locked myself in the bathroom. As I looked in the mirror, all I could think was, *It's not a spider bite. He didn't answer the question about leukemia. It's not good that it didn't hurt. He's talking to my uncle... It's bad... I have cancer.* I looked at the lump, examining it again while crying, wishing it hurt.

"You took her to an Urgent Care doctor? What the fuck does an Urgent Care doctor know?" We were back at my uncle's house, and I could hear my Aunt Susan on the other end of the phone talking as my uncle walked over to me.

"It's Susan," my uncle said as he handed me the phone.

"Hi, Aunt Susan," I said with an upbeat voice, not knowing what she had heard.

"Hi, I understand Uncle David took you to an Urgent Care doctor. I'm sorry, but what the fuck does an Urgent Care doctor know. On Monday, I'll take you to a real doctor. Dr. Greaney is my doctor, and he is fabulous," she said.

"Okay, that sounds good. Thank you, Aunt Susan," I said as I wiped away the tears.

CHAPTER NINE

Boyfriend

"John, it's Joy. I found a lump on my throat, I saw a doctor, and I think I have cancer. So… give me a call when you get a chance." This was the message I left, which was punctuated with sniffles and pregnant pauses. It was Thanksgiving, and he was with his mom. I pictured him calling me back as soon as he got the message, coming over to see me, and giving me a big hug to comfort me. That's what happens in the movies, so I assumed that's what would happen in real life. I mean, I made him "so happy" so…. he should be calling any second now. Any second…

Friday

No call back... sniffle.

Saturday

Not a word... sniffle, sniffle.

Sunday

Seriously?

Monday

What the bleep?!

Tuesday

Maybe he's dead?

Not exactly the reaction I was expecting, but maybe he was dead and unable to call me, I mean it was plausible. Let's not assume the worst. The worst being that he was alive and well and not calling me back. Okay, the dead thing is technically the worse of the two, but come on.

I had tests done, and by Tuesday I had the results of my chest x-ray and lump aspiration. The news was not good. My chest x-ray lit up like a Christmas tree, and my aspiration results confirmed that I had cancer. "That's why you've been coughing so much," my oncologist said to me. "The tumors have been making you cough."

"Oh, wow." I couldn't believe it was that bad.

"It's in two different places above your diaphragm, so it's still considered to be stage two. It's most likely Hodgkin's lymphoma, but we need to wait for the biopsy results. Hodgkin's lymphoma is actually what we're hoping for. It has a higher success rate than non-Hodgkin's lymphoma, and it's easier to treat," she informed me.

Next, I found out I would have to go through chemotherapy. "What happens if I don't do the chemotherapy?" I asked.

"You'll be dead within the year."

My aunt and I kept our fingers crossed that I had what I started to refer to as "the good kind of cancer."

I wanted to talk to John, to tell him what was happening, how I felt, and for him to comfort me. I knew he was visiting his mom. Maybe something happened that kept him from checking his voicemail, like perhaps he was dead. Then I would feel horrible for being mad at him for not calling me back. My troubles were nothing compared to his. Maybe he was mangled in a hospital somewhere. Once again, I was the lucky one here. I mean there had to be an explanation as to why he hadn't returned my call. Why else would he not call me back after a message like that?

So I called him, but this time I called him from my aunt's phone. She had a phone number that came up as unlisted in caller ID, and this time... he answered.

"This is John."

"Hi, this is Joy."

"Click."

He hung up on me! He was not dead! The only reasonable explanation besides an alien abduction went out the window.

When I hung up the phone… after he hung up the phone… I was SO angry! How could he? What a jerk! Who would do that to someone? My heart beat loudly, I could hear it in my ears, and then I felt it, a pain in the lump on my neck, the same lump that hadn't hurt at all before. I put my hand on it and started to calm down. It was one of those moments in life when you don't calm down because you are in a relaxing environment, but because you know that your life depends on it.

In that moment I thought of my favorite motivational speaker, Zig Ziglar. He told a story about being stuck in an airport, and all he wanted to do was go home. He waited in line to check in, and when he finally got to the person behind the counter, she told him his flight had been canceled. Instead of getting upset or mad, he looked at her and said, "Fantastic!" He wasn't going to let this situation ruin his day. He thought of all of the reasons why it was good that his flight had been canceled and recognized that he was fortunate enough to be in a nice warm airport where he could get some important work done. The best part was that at the end of his story, he added that people always asked, "Now Zig, I've heard of those positive thinkers, but come on, did you really feel that way?"

He responded, "Well, of course not! At least not initially." He went on to say, "They can cancel my flight, but they can not cancel my day. You see, the day is mine, given to me by the Lord himself." This story always shifted my perspective on how to look at things.

I thought, *If Zig can do that with his flight being canceled, then I can do that with cancer.* That is when I stopped looking at the negatives in my life and I started looking at the positives, and as unbelievable as it sounds I had a ton of positives.

"I'm grateful that I found the lump because if I hadn't I wouldn't know that I have cancer and I wouldn't be getting treatment for it. I'm grateful to my uncle for taking me to Urgent Care because if I hadn't gone, I wouldn't know that I have cancer and I wouldn't be able to treat it. I'm grateful to my aunt for taking care of me and taking me to my appointments and introducing me to a great doctor. I'm grateful for all of my friends and family who have been sending me their love and support."

I had my list of reasons why I was grateful that I found out I had cancer. It's amazing how much this helped me change my perspective. Of course, I still had my moments of "why me?" but saying all of the positive things out loud every day really helped relieve some of the stress I was feeling. I was so grateful that I had listened to Zig's motivational speeches before I got sick.

A week later I received a phone call from a number I didn't recognize.

"Hello," I said as I answered the phone.

"Is this Joy?" a voice on the line asked.

"Yes, this is she."

"Oh, yeah. Hi, this is John's friend. John wanted me to tell you that he doesn't want to see you ever again and that you were a bitch and that things just weren't working out," he said.

"Are you kidding me?" I asked. I couldn't believe he was doing this, but I had no control over what he was doing or what his friend was saying to me. I did have control over my actions, so I pulled the phone away from my ear as his friend continued to say horrible things, and I pressed the end call button. I was in survival mode, and this was not anything I had time or energy to deal with. I was fighting for my life.

"I'm grateful that I found out I have cancer and discovered what kind of a person John is. Thank you, God. I mean you could have found a different way of telling me, but thank you." If God were to respond, it would be something like this, "Well, I did have someone actually TELL

47

you that you should stay away from him. It didn't work. I had to go up a level, and you're welcome." I picture God to be funny and a bit sassy.

CHAPTER TEN

Reactions

When I called my friends at SeaWorld, I distinctly remember two reactions. One was from my friend, Christine, the girl who was hired at the same time I was, and the other was from Ann. When I got done telling Christine, she asked, "Do you want me to tell anyone?" I paused for a moment.

"Yeah, tell anyone who cares. If there is ever a time that I need my friends, it's now."

With that Christine mobilized the SeaWorld training department to support me. People were arranging which days they could cover to travel the three plus hours to Ventura to spend time with me.

It was like a black and white cartoon where a tower pops up and Morse code beeps went out over SeaWorld, letting everyone know that one of their own needed help.

There was one person named Hoppi who contacted me from SeaWorld. I didn't know Hoppi, but we had something in common: cancer. He had just survived Hodgkin's lymphoma and took me under his wing to guide me. He drove up to Ventura, a three-hour drive, to spend time with me and answer all of my questions. Once again, I had never met him before this moment. This was just one example of the heart these people had. They would do anything for the animals and anything for one of their own.

The other reaction that I distinctly remember was Ann's. I called to tell her what happened and that I had cancer. I told her about the lump and the x-ray that confirmed it. I told her about how I would have to go through chemotherapy. At the end of me spilling every detail to her over the phone, probably a good ten minutes, I stopped to hear what she had to say.

"I'm sorry. What?" she asked.

"Ann, are you serious?"

"Yes. What did you just say?"

"Ann, are you kidding me?" I said, kind of annoyed that she was saying this after I poured my heart out to her.

"I'm sorry. It's just that after you said the word *cancer* I couldn't hear you anymore. I couldn't hear anything. Everything just stopped," she said. "So, if you would be so kind as to start from the beginning and tell me again what has happened - I need to understand what is happening," she said with a soft and shaky voice.

It hadn't occurred to me that this was not just happening to me, but it was happening to everyone in my life who loved me. Ann's reaction embodied the surreal moment of finding out that your friend has cancer.

CHAPTER ELEVEN

Goodbye, Film School

"You're telling me that I can't just attend the classes and learn, but not do the film shoots?" I asked my film school over the phone.

"Yes, you have to do both at the same time," the cold female voice said from the other end of the phone.

"But I just found out that I have cancer, and I have to go through chemotherapy. I'm going to be exhausted and unable to do the shoots, but I still want to learn. I want to go to the classes and learn," I pleaded with the less than caring voice. I mean, you'd think I would have some sort of a cancer card to play here. Maybe they would be somewhat sympathetic… but no, that was not the case.

"There is no way that we can allow you to only go to the classes."

"I understand if you don't give me credit. That's fine, but I still want to learn. I wasn't expecting to get cancer. I didn't think it would be a problem to just go to class to learn." In reality, I thought they would be very supportive. The effort to still learn should have been commended.

"I'm sorry. There is nothing I can do," she said. I hung up the phone and sat in silence in my car in the school parking lot. It was dark already, and all I could hear was silence as I stared back at the school. My life had completely gone off track. CUT TO BLACK.

Then I did what any filmmaker would do, I turned to the movies to ease my mind. I rented all of these movies that had a main character with cancer. Guess what I saw? All of these people who died in the end - this wasn't exactly helpful. Plus, I knew that there were millions of cancer survivors out there. Where were their stories?

I couldn't believe that film school had said, "No," to me returning to learn. It seemed so absurd that they would stop me.

That's when a fleeting thought in the background became more and more real. *I could make a documentary on myself and show a story of survival. That way I could still learn about filmmaking.* My aunt mentioned it to me one day while we were on our way to one of my appointments. "Have you thought about making a documentary on what you are going through?" she asked.

"I've actually thought about it. I'm not sure though," I replied, but the seed had been planted.

After Thanksgiving break I went in to say goodbye to my film teacher and to let him know why I wouldn't be back. He just had a look of shock and didn't quite know what to say.

As I walked out of the classroom I passed by my desk and thought about the moment when the students would return to class and occupy their desks to learn about filmmaking, while my desk would remain empty. It felt like I had dropped off the face of the planet.

As I started to walk out of the school, I decided to stop by equipment checkout to see if Ellis was there.

"Hey, what can I help you with?" Ellis asked as I walked in.

"Well, I came in to say goodbye. I found out that I have cancer, and I have to drop out," I said.

"What? Oh, Joy, I'm so sorry."

"It's okay, I'll be okay," I said, reassuring myself at the same time.

"Let me know if I can do anything for you."

"Actually, I do have something. Do you think you could come with me to film my first chemotherapy treatment?"

"Yes, absolutely. I'll be there. Are you planning to make a documentary?"

"Actually, yes. The school said I can't continue my classes, so I figure if I can't learn at film school, then I can learn while making a documentary on myself," I said with a smile and a new sense of determination. "Also, have you noticed that every film about cancer has the person dying in the end? It's awful. There are so many survivors out there. I want to show a story of survival."

"Wait, what? They said you *can't* keep taking your classes?"

"That's right."

"What?"

"I know."

"Well, the documentary sounds amazing. I'm in," he said as he looked at me with a newly found admiration.

"Thanks Ellis, my first chemotherapy is Monday at 8 a.m. in Ventura. Do you think you can make it?"

"Wouldn't miss it for the world."

Over the weekend I got a call from Ellis. "Hey, I have a group of guys here who want to show their support by shaving their heads."

"What? Really? Who?" I asked in disbelief.

"Just a bunch of guys who think it stinks that you have to go through this. I'll film it if you want. All you have to do is be here to shave their heads."

When I walked in the classroom where I had my first film class, there were about six guys who I barely knew waiting there and Mr. Schwartz, my first teacher at film school, who had heard about it and stayed to watch and show his support. Some of the guys I recognized from equipment checkout, but there were others who I didn't know at all. I had only been at film school a short time and didn't know many people.

"Oh my gosh! I can't believe you guys are doing this. Thank you so much," I said.

"Of course! We're sorry you have to go through this," one guy said. They were all so nice and humble.

"Here you go," Ellis said as he handed me the clippers.

"I've never used clippers before. Can you do it for a little bit?" I asked. The guy who was sitting in the chair, ready to get his hair buzzed, cringed in nervous anticipation.

"Sure," Ellis said. With that he started to shave this guy's hair off. Then it was my turn. I was laughing and coughing while shaving their heads. At one point there was a weird noise with the clippers while I was shaving one person's head. My heart dropped. I pulled the clippers away from his head and looked at his face.

"Oh my gosh! Are you okay?" I asked with a look of horror. I was certain that I had cut off an ear or lacerated his head.

"I'm okay. I'm okay," he said chuckling at my reaction. I laughed too as I looked back at his head to make sure that everything was still there.

It was an incredibly sweet gesture by people who barely knew me.

"Thank you, God, for showing me all of the good people who are in this world," I said to myself. I had found a new reason to be grateful.

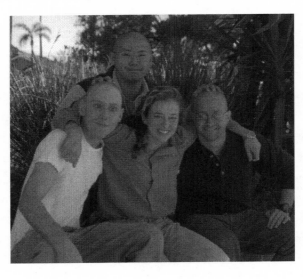

CHAPTER TWELVE

First Chemotherapy

On my first day of chemotherapy I was so nervous that I fainted. I walked into the bathroom at my aunt's house, closed the door, then started to notice that my vision was narrowing and getting darker. Luckily I knew what was happening. I lowered myself down to the ground so I wouldn't fall and hit my head. The next thing I knew I was looking at the ceiling of the bathroom. There was no reason to faint, except for the fact that I was getting ready for my 8:00 a.m. appointment to receive my first dose of chemotherapy.

Hoppi told me to bring candies to suck on because sometimes you can taste the chemo. As he told me this, his face puckered up just thinking about the taste. "Bring headphones so you can listen to relaxing music and make sure they use different veins. When they stick to one vein, it can ruin it, so try rotating which vein they use," he told me.

This was all good information, but it may have contributed to elevated nerves. Of course, there was also my limited knowledge of what happens during chemotherapy, which was filled in with images from movies and television shows. From this bastion of knowledge I was able to figure out that people throw up after chemotherapy. It was always over-dramatically portrayed that the cancer patient was curled up next to the toilet after their chemotherapy treatment.

So, I suppose I had good reason to faint. When my aunt and I reached the hospital, we happened to get into the elevator with my oncologist. I turned to her and said, "I was so nervous about my first chemo treatment that I fainted this morning." She looked at me and then back to the doors of the elevator. She smiled and nodded slightly. THAT WAS IT! That was her compassionate response. That was the response of my doctor who was supposed to care in some way about me, or at least that was what I believed a good doctor should do. I was, after all, putting my life in her hands. A simple, "It will be okay," would have been just fine, but no response was just unimaginable. The doors to the elevator opened and she took the opportunity to exit immediately.

"That was strange," my aunt said. Then she exited the elevator.

"Yes, it was," I said.

I did not exit. I just stood there because part of me wanted to let the doors close, return to the first floor, get in my car, and get the heck out of there. But, I couldn't do that because then I would be dead within the year (also, my aunt had the car keys). *All right, Joy, you can do this. You are stronger than this. Let's go kill it!* I said to myself. Then my feet started to move, and I exited the elevator.

I had to remember that I was lucky. My biopsy results had come back as Hodgkin's lymphoma, THE GOOD KIND OF CANCER! Yes, I was going through chemotherapy, but my chances of survival were high. Everything would be okay. It was another thing to be grateful for.

"Did I miss anything?" Ellis asked as he walked into the waiting room with his camera.

"No, I just checked in," I said.

"Joy," a nurse called for me. It was go time. They took me back to get a finger prick blood sample. They needed to make sure I had enough white blood cells to be able to get the treatment. My levels were fine, so they had me go into another room with cozy chairs.

"Oh, this is nice," I said as the nurse escorted me to my very own comfy chair.

"Are you nervous?" Ellis asked.

"Yes, but it's okay. I've got a CD player to listen to with my favorite songs."

As the nurse worked on getting my chemo ready, I pulled out my mints, CD player, and headphones. She brought a metal table over with everything she needed to give me an IV. I had already been poked and prodded, so I knew that some nurses got the stick right away and others did not. Sometimes they would miss the vein then search for it under the skin with the needle. That was the worst.

"Are you pretty good at this?" I asked with a smile, but I really wanted to know.

"Well, I've been doing this a long time," she said as she prepared all of the equipment on the metal table for me.

"So, what should I expect to feel after getting my treatment?" I asked.

"It's all on those sheets the doctor gave you."

"Sheets?" I asked.

"Didn't the doctor give you that information? It's on one page sheets that explains what to expect with each chemotherapy."

"No," I replied, realizing that I disliked my doctor even more now.

I was clearly just a number to this oncologist. I was not twenty-five year old Joy Christiana Clausen. I was a number, and she did not care if I lived or died or if I fainted from nerves before my chemotherapy. She couldn't even be bothered to give me information on the side effects I should expect. Just then the door opened and my friend, Kevin walked in. Ellis was standing behind a tripod filming me, and I had just taken out my camera to get some close ups of my arm.

"I'm so sorry I'm late," he said.

"I wasn't going to say that on tape, Kevin," I said as I filmed him and then panned over to the IV in my arm.

"But, thank you," I said.

Kevin was someone I met at film school. I barely knew him. We went to one movie together, but the second he heard about what happened he was there for me. He had just experienced his grandmother dying of liver cancer the previous year. When he heard that I was diagnosed with cancer, he wanted to help someone who was still so young try to win her battle.

He wrote me a letter of encouragement:

> I know that it's finally starting to sink in that you are beginning a battle that will probably be one of the greatest challenges in your life that you will ever have to face. This is an illness that has to be fought 30% physically and 70% mentally. There is no other alternative but to win this battle. If you start to feel weak-hearted, let me know. I'll be there to cheer you on and give you the encouragement that you need. Sometimes you just need a friend. I can't fight the fight for you, Joy, but I can be your coach.

It was so nice knowing that I had someone in my corner helping me fight.

"This might feel a little cold when it goes in your veins. Let me know if you feel any discomfort," the nurse said as she got ready to start my chemotherapy.

"Okay. Can I put my headphones on before you start?" I asked.

"Oh, sure."

I put my headphones on and listened to my favorite music and pictured myself surrounded by warm healing sunlight. The song "I Can See Clearly Now" came on.

JOY CLAUSEN SOTO

I Can See Clearly Now

I can see clearly now, the rain is gone,
I can see all obstacles in my way
Gone are the dark clouds that had me blind
It's gonna be a bright (bright), bright (bright) Sun-Shiny day.
I think I can make it now, the pain is gone
All of the bad feelings have disappeared
Here is the rainbow I've been prayin for
It's gonna be a bright (bright), bright (bright) Sun-Shiny day.
Look all around, there's nothing but blue skies
Look straight ahead, nothing but blue skies
I can see clearly now, the rain is gone,
I can see all obstacles in my way
Gone are the dark clouds that had me blind
It's gonna be a bright (bright), bright (bright) Sun-Shiny day.

—Johnny Nash

CHAPTER THIRTEEN

"For Some Reason..."

"Hi, I need you to call the office when you have a chance," my oncologist said in a voicemail. My blood went cold. *Why would she be calling me?* I thought. Doctors don't call patients normally.

I had just finished watching *The Lord of the Rings* in the theater with Kevin and another friend from film school. Earlier that day I had my second round of chemotherapy, and they were both by my side the entire time. The truth was I felt fine. Yes, I just finished having a bunch of chemicals designed to destroy the cancer that was killing me pumped into my body. Yes, these chemicals had a lot of side effects, but I just didn't feel that bad. I still had my hair. I wasn't throwing up. I felt normal with the exception of the occasional realization that I was fighting for my life and the fact that everyone was being REALLY nice to me. I was simply a girl at the movies with her friends having a great time.

I saw the missed call as we walked back to Kevin's red Camaro after the movie. A slight chill went down my back when I heard the message. Hands down, in an instant you know something is wrong when your doctor leaves you a message. "Why," you ask? Because

THE DOCTOR is calling! Doctor's don't make calls. Their assistants do. Doctors don't call to reschedule or to say that you had a great pap smear. A doctor calls because something isn't right. I told my friends that it was the doctor and that I was worried. They tried to reassure me that it was nothing, but I had a sinking feeling. The next day I reached my oncologist.

"I'm sorry. What?" I asked my oncologist over the phone.

"It looks like your slides were sent to Stanford... for some reason," she said. I got stuck on the "for some reason" part. You're my doctor, and you don't know why my slides were sent there? Why didn't you send them there yourself? Those words, "... for some reason" kept ringing in my head, but there was more information that I needed to hear. "Stanford is like the mecca for lymphomas, and they said it is actually large B cell non-Hodgkin's lymphoma." My heart dropped. It was the kind of cancer that we didn't want to have.

"So what does that mean now? I just finished my second round of chemotherapy," I said.

"Yeah, I know. We're going to have to adjust your chemotherapy protocol. It's going to be a more aggressive treatment."

As soon as I got home, I walked into my aunt's bedroom crying.

"I just got a call from the doctor. She said that, *for some reason*, my slides were sent to Stanford and that I actually have non-Hodgkin's lymphoma," I said while sobbing.

"What, Joy? She said what?" she asked. I don't communicate well when I'm crying. It comes out as gibberish.

"I actually have non-Hodgkin's lymphoma," I said as I took a breath and tried to communicate in a way where I could be understood. Aunt Susan hugged me, and I could hear her sniffling.

"I know. I'll call Dr. Siegel," she said. Aunt Susan always knew what to do. There was always a solution to any problem, and if she didn't have the solution, she knew who did, and she knew how to contact them.

"Who?" I asked. She was already looking through her phone book and had picked up the phone to dial.

"Dr. Siegel. He is incredible. He'll know what to do." Now, I don't know how she got a hold of him on her first try, but she did. Soon she was speaking directly to him. "Hi, Dr. Siegel. We need your help. My niece Joy just found out that she has a different type of cancer...." and with that she broke down, and for the first time in my life I saw my Aunt Susan cry. When I saw this, I immediately stopped crying, and this will sound bizarre, but I thought, *WOW, she really loves me.* She regained her composure because she is Aunt Susan, and she is amazing. "We need your help. Can you help us?" she asked with a shaky voice. When she got off the phone, she said, "Okay, he is going to have his head pathologist look at your slides. We just need to drive them down to Children's Hospital in Los Angeles tomorrow."

If Dr. Siegel confirmed that it was non-Hodgkin's lymphoma, then it meant a few things. One, I was up for a much bigger battle. Two, I had no trust in my doctor who didn't even know why my slides were sent out in the first place. Three, if divine intervention hadn't taken place, and some random person hadn't sent in those slides, I would have been under-treated for my cancer, and my chances of survival would have plummeted.

"Eggnog and bourbon?" my aunt asked me. It was December after all. "Uhhh..."

"I say we get drunk," she said.

"Sure, I'll have an eggnog and bourbon. Is it bourbon or rum?"

"It's bourbon," she said and turned around to make us some drinks. She brought the spiked eggnogs up to her bedroom, and we watched a movie while sipping on the drinks. I have to say it was a particularly strong drink, and I didn't think it was the best idea that I was having it, so I just had a sip, and that was it. During the movie she turned to me with a mischievous smile and asked, "Are you as drunk as I am?"

"Oh yeah," I said even though I wasn't drunk at all. I didn't want to break that magical moment with her. We sat in bed watching a movie while we bonded over eggnog and a cancer misdiagnosis.

"Thank you, God, for these wonderful moments with Aunt Susan."

CHAPTER FOURTEEN

The Waiting Game

The waiting game began. We dropped off my slides at Children's Hospital Los Angeles (CHLA) on Friday. Did I mention it was Friday, December 21st? It was the holidays, not an ideal situation for my sanity. I had to wait until the following Wednesday to find out if it was definitely non-Hodgkin's lymphoma. This is when I entered a mental battle with myself.

During all of this my aunt was getting ready for her wedding. She had set the date to get married on Saturday, December 29th. Her house was full of people. Her fiancé, his children, and their children were in the house, not to mention the poor niece with cancer (that would be me).

My mom flew out for the wedding. She had wanted to fly out earlier to be with me after I found out I had cancer, but I told her I was okay, and she didn't have to come out.

I know this sounds weird, but when I was growing up I noticed that people would get distracted when my mom walked in the room. One time when I had my braces put on, my mom walked in at the very end to see how I was doing. We went home afterward and as the week went on, the pain in my mouth kept getting worse and worse. Finally, my mom took me back to the orthodontist, who saw exactly what was wrong when I opened my mouth. He had forgotten to cut all of the wires on my braces. I had long wires rubbing up against the back of my mouth every time I tried to eat or talk. The minute I heard that I knew why. It was because my mom had come in to check on me when the orthodontist was almost done installing my braces. My mom was a very pretty woman, who used to be a model. I saw the way men looked at her. They got all weird and goofy and distracted. That is how the orthodontist acted when she walked in the room. That's why I knew he had forgotten because she walked in the room.

When I found out I had cancer, I didn't want her to distract people. I didn't want anyone to make mistakes, and I didn't want to take care of her. I always felt as if I had to protect her and keep her safe. I knew that she would be so upset by this, and I didn't want to have to pick her up or tell her it would be okay. I needed to be the one who was picked up and told it was going to be okay. I wanted to be surrounded by people who didn't cry when they looked at me. I felt awful about it, but I needed to do what was best for me.

CHAPTER FIFTEEN

One Percent

Let's not forget that I was still making a documentary with the hope of showing a story of survival. Finding out that it was a more aggressive cancer was not good news for the outcome, but I still wanted to document everything. I went upstairs in my aunt's house and recorded a video diary. It was cathartic to record these moments. I was able to get out the emotions that I couldn't share with other people. The camera became my confidant.

VIDEO DIARY: December 22nd, 2001

*I'm feeling okay right now physically, but I don't feel very good mentally. I feel much better than I did yesterday because I know that **if one percent of people get through this, that's going to be me. I'm going to get through this**. It just kind of sucked to hear different news than what I thought. I thought I was fighting one thing, and now I'm fighting another, but regardless, I'm going to win. That's what I'm here to tell you right now, my video journal. Drinking soda water helps. I would* *like some Ginger Ale, but I don't know if we have any in the house. Last night I threw up, not because I really had to, but because I wanted to throw up. You know that feeling you get when you want to throw up and it would feel so good if you could? Well, you should keep everything down in your stomach, which really does make sense, but I didn't do it because I just wanted it to be out so badly.*

But, I'm doing better today. I'm getting calls from everyone. They're going to do a prayer service thing on the Internet where they get a lot of people to pray and think about me at the same time. So, all of these really nice things are happening. Once again you realize how much people care and how good people are when something like this happens. It brings out the best in people or the worst in people, and you get to see that aspect. It's really, really nice to see. I'm glad that I'm getting to see this from everyone, and I'm glad that I get to know how much people love me and care about me. A lot of times they'll probably see me or hear me crying over the phone when they say something nice, but it's because I'm just so happy about it. It's tears of joy, tears of happiness. That's about it for today. I will see you next time I feel well enough to do this.

CHAPTER SIXTEEN

Send Me Your Pain

"The second opinion came back. It's the bad kind, Ann," I said through tears. I was walking back to my hotel room to get ready for my aunt's wedding.

"Okay, what does this mean?" she asked.

"It means a lot more chemotherapy, and now I have a lower chance of surviving." I just couldn't believe it. How did this happen? I arrived at my hotel room. "Ann, I've got to go. I'll talk to you later."

"We are going to get through this, Joy."

"Okay."

I was alone in my hotel room, and the full weight of what was happening hit me. On top of that I was bloated, constipated, weak, and losing my hair in clumps.

I turned on the camera and unleashed all of my feelings. What came out was Mount-Everest-climbing-Joy versus scared-Joy in a battle to remain positive.

VIDEO DIARY: December 28th, 2001

All right... my hair started falling out yesterday. So, I got it all cut off (in a bob style) and I like it a lot. I'm going to get it done right now for the wedding, but God I've been feeling so sorry for myself it's unbelievable. It's so bad, and it's making the cancer grow because I'm upset, and I want to stop.

AHHHH. I don't want to be like this. I don't want to be feeling sorry for myself, BUT I AM. So, I'm going to go downstairs and get my hair done for the wedding and stop feeling sorry for myself and carry my head up high and... smile, but my hair is falling out. GOOD TIMES! No more hair for Joy. The bald look is in.

My stomach goes on and off with feeling sour. Like right now it feels sour. But, yeah, I'm pretty much feeling sorry for myself right now. So, I need to stop that!

Okay, so suck it up. Suck it up. So, next time you see me, I'm going to be pretty.

My nose is bleeding, and I feel like crap, but it's because I'm making myself feel like crap because I'm feeling sorry for myself, so STOP IT! Ahhhhhhhhh! A battle of the wills! Stop it! Okay. God! Stop feeling sorry for yourself! There's no reason. People go through stuff all the time. Stop it! I'm such a lucky person to have all the people who love me and to have done all the stuff that I've done in my life. I'm just too lucky, so, sooo lucky to be feeling like this. I've got to stop. Stop it. Okay. I'm going to go now. I'll be pretty. Okay, bye, bye.

I'm going to win. I'm going to win.

After I turned off the camera and took some deep breaths, I saw that I missed a call from Ann. This was her voicemail:

"Joy, I just don't know how one person can handle all of the pain that you are going through. So, I was thinking that if you could send me some of your pain, if we could split it up between the two of us, it would be easier for you. So, if you wouldn't mind, please send me your pain. I'll be waiting. I love you."

It was exactly what I needed to hear. Of course I couldn't send her my pain, but just knowing that I had a friend who was willing to take it from me meant so much. The fact that she thought about this and sincerely wanted to take my pain was just unbelievable. I may have been in a mental battle, but hearing my friend's message during my darkest hour helped take me out of my head. I called her afterward.

"Ann, I have no idea how you knew what I was going through just now, but thank you so much for your message. I love you."

That's what you will find out about cancer. It can bring out different things in different people. I was lucky enough to have a best friend with a pure heart who wanted to walk through the fire with me. For that I will be eternally grateful.

"Thank you, God, for my wonderful friends!"

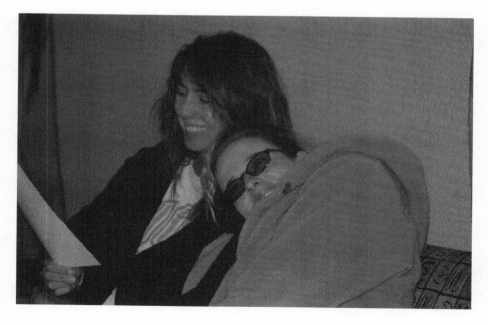

CHAPTER SEVENTEEN

Sneakers at a Wedding

VIDEO DIARY: December 30th, 2001

Hello, it's me. It's the next day after the wedding, and I'm feeling pretty good right now. I'm winning! Yes, I'm winning right now. I'm feeling pretty good physically and emotionally. I'm going downstairs right now, and I'm going to eat breakfast with my family, but my hair is still falling out. As short as it is, it's still falling out.

Just wanted to update you. I was losing the fight yesterday, but today I'm winning it. That's how it's going to be I think, day-by-day, winning and losing, and I'm going to come out on top.

Yesterday was a bad day.

I'm winning, I'm winning, I'm happy. It's going well. It's day-by-day. You have to learn this if you ever go through anything like this. If you know anyone who goes through cancer or anything else life threatening, treat him or her like a human being. Don't feel sorry for them. Don't let them see you feel sorry for them because I'll tell you if I see that in someone's eyes, I'm done. I can't do it. I start crying.

I danced last night at the wedding, and when I was dancing, I felt so much better. It just took my mind off of not feeling good. The endorphins kicked in, and I felt good last night. I need to get out and do more things so I'm not just feeling sorry for myself like I was for the past couple of days.

I saw Dr. Greaney (my aunt's doctor) at the wedding last night, and he made me feel a lot better about everything. I was upstairs in a room hibernating by myself, and he came up and talked to me for a while and tried to convince me to come downstairs. I said, 'I don't want to go downstairs because the shoes I have, which aren't mine, are really wobbly and so I'm falling all over the place in them.'

He said, "Well..." looking across the room and seeing my sneakers, "I'd like to see you in those sneakers."

So, I wore a very nice outfit and SNEAKERS. I went downstairs and danced the night away in my sneakers. That was fun, I had a good time.

He said, 'You know what? People are usually about 85 when they realize they can do whatever they want to do, and it doesn't matter because they shouldn't care what other people think and you, having a life threatening illness at 25, realize that now.'

So, I'm feeling much better. Live life to the fullest. Who cares? You only get one life, right? All right, that's about it. Bye-bye.

CHAPTER EIGHTEEN

New Hairstyle

"Hey, can you shave my head today?" I asked my brother.

"Sure," he responded quietly.

I wanted someone special to shave my head and someone who had experience with clippers. The last thing I wanted was to hear the sound I heard when I shaved that guy's head at film school.

"Hey, Ellis, I'm shaving my head today. Can you film it?" I asked over the phone. I was still making a documentary, and I knew that this would be important footage to get.

"Absolutely. Do you need me to get anything?" he asked.

"No, I think we have everything, thanks." Ellis came over and set up his camera in the bathroom while my brother and I waited. I put some dark, red lipstick on to help me look more feminine after all of my hair came off.

"Whenever you're ready," Ellis said after setting up his camera.

"Okay, let's do this." I clapped my hands together to get everyone psyched. Okay, mainly to get myself psyched. My brother turned on the clippers, which made a horrid, electric buzzing sound when they were powered on. "Bzzzzzzzz," the electric clippers got closer to my head. My brother wasn't going slowly with them either. *Too fast, too fast!* I thought. I moved my head away to safety. My brother turned the clippers off.

"Do you want me to do it or...?" he asked.

"Okay, just do it really slowly."

He turned the clippers on again, and this time I didn't move. In the mirror I could see hair, lots of hair, falling to the ground. The good part was that I couldn't see my bald scalp at first, so it wasn't that bad. I stood there in the bathroom with a smile on my face as I looked in the mirror. In all honesty the smile was for the camera. I didn't want it to look like it was that bad.

"Bzzzzzzz," more hair fell to the ground, and my smile started to quiver. I could see my scalp now. Reality was setting in. Then tears started to drip down my face. "All right, you guys have to... make me laugh," I said through tears.

Ellis let out a long sigh, "Hmmmmm."

No one said anything, because let's face it... what in the world could they say?

Then my brother asked, "Do you want me to leave your sideburns?"

"Yeah, I want to get rid..." I started to reply in a high-pitched voice through tears and laughter.

He then asked, "You want to get rid of them or leave them?"

"Yeah! No! Get rid of them! Who leaves their sideburns?" I asked him still laughing and wiping away my tears.

He put his hand on my shoulder and with a loving smile said, "I told you I'd make you laugh." He turned an extremely difficult moment into a beautiful one between a brother and a sister.

The next day I played with my new look. My aunt had taken me wig shopping after I found out I had cancer and some friends gave me wigs and caps, so I was prepared for this moment. I tried on my auburn wig, two blonde wigs, a scarf, and a warm blue hat. Apparently I had different personalities with the different looks. According to Kevin I was a lot nicer when I wore the blonde wigs and a little bitchy when I wore the auburn wig. Note taken.

"So, I did it. I shaved my head," I told my step-mom over the phone.

"Oh, sweetie. How do you feel?" she asked.

"Well, it changes things because now I look like a cancer patient. It feels more real now," I said.

"Oh, I know, sweetie, and then when your eyebrows and eyelashes fall out, that stinks too," she said.

Wait, what? Backup a smidge.

"I'm sorry, what?" I asked.

"Yeah, you didn't know that? Your eyebrows and eyelashes fall out too at some point, but I don't think it's until later." Wait a minute... I didn't sign up for a naked face. I might look like an alien and with the wigs I would either be a bitchy alien or a nice alien. Oh man.

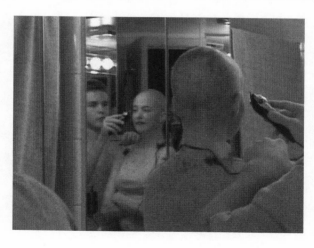

CHAPTER NINETEEN

"Battle!"

"You have to be ready for BATTLE!"

I was having a tough time after my diagnosis changed. I personified defeat. My shoulders slouched, and my head hung low. My aunt thought that Dr. Greaney could help. He was the same doctor who gave me a pep talk at her wedding and got me to dance in my sneakers. He was the primary care physician that my aunt wanted me to see, or maybe I should say the "real doctor" she wanted me to see instead of the Urgent Care doctor. Unfortunately, he had been out of the office the first half of the week so I wasn't able to see him until after it was confirmed that I had cancer. Dr. Greaney had an Irish accent, dark brown hair, and a thick mustache.

My aunt and I walked into his office, although for me it was more of a shuffle than a walk. Surely he was going to tell me that things weren't that bad, tell me why I should be able to survive this, read some statistics. Instead something else happened.

"You are preparing to go into battle. This is war you are going into, and you need to be prepared. You have to be ready for battle! I am your

General, and your oncologist is your Lieutenant, and we will devise a plan of how to win this war. You are not alone in this battle." Then he looked at me, clenched his fist and said, "Battle! Battle! Battle!"

What was happening? This was the weirdest and most wonderful speech I could ever receive from a doctor. It was as if I was getting a speech straight out of the movie, *Braveheart*. Somehow this helped me feel as though I had some sort of control over the situation. I was going into battle, and I would fight. I walked, nay, marched out of his office. My shoulders back, my head held high. I only saw him a few times more, but he had done his job. He prepared my mind and spirit for what was ahead. I was ready to take on the world, and most importantly, I was ready for my "battle" with cancer.

CHAPTER TWENTY

Dr. Siegel

Dr. Siegel, the oncologist at Children's Hospital Los Angeles, was nothing like my oncologist in Ventura. He was nice and took the time to explain my cancer and treatment to me. Most importantly, he treated me like a person, not a number. My other oncologist couldn't even talk to me like a human being in the elevator that day after I told her I was so nervous that I passed out. Unfortunately, Dr. Siegel was not my oncologist. He was simply giving a second opinion.

He sent his treatment recommendation to her office. I was so happy that I had a plan from a doctor I felt like I could trust with my life. Then I spoke to my oncologist on the phone. "We can't do this. No hospital here will administer this treatment," she said.

"Why not?" I asked in disbelief, while trying to remain calm.

"It's a very aggressive treatment, and no one here has experience giving this to adults. It's a pediatric protocol. I spoke to several hospitals here, and they all said they won't do it," she said.

I didn't know what to do. I wanted to go with the treatment he recommended. He was the person I trusted. I didn't even want to hear what my other oncologist had to say because at that point I had lost all trust in her.

Later that week I had an appointment set up to meet with Dr. Siegel to go over the treatment plan and answer any questions. As Aunt Susan and I walked up to Children's Hospital Los Angeles, we passed by giant children's blocks outside that spelled out CHLA. The big glass doors opened, and I saw these large glass windows on the right that let in so much light. There was a play area for kids and big works of art made for children. I felt lighter just walking in, as if I were safe.

Aunt Susan and I waited for Dr. Siegel in an exam room. It was a normal exam room, but when I looked up, I spotted hand painted butterflies on the ceiling tiles. There was a knock at the door, and Dr. Siegel walked in. He had gray hair and wore a white lab coat with one side of his lapel overflowing with colorful pins. He listened to all of my questions and took the time to give me thorough answers. I felt like his only patient. I felt like he cared about me.

"I'm recommending a more aggressive therapy to make sure we kill all of the cancer cells that may be hiding in your body," he said. This involved overnight hospital stays while I received chemotherapy and spinal taps at the beginning and end of each treatment. For the spinal taps they would take out some spinal fluid and then inject me with chemotherapy to make sure they were killing everything.

He let me know it was a tougher treatment, but that they had experienced great success with it and my type of cancer. Since I was younger, my body could handle more chemotherapy, and I had a better chance of being cured.

"Now, I understand that your doctors in Ventura aren't familiar with this method so I met with the hospital board and received approval to have you treated here," he said.

"What? Really? I get to be treated here? That's incredible!" I said as I felt tears well up in my eyes. "Thank you so much! Will you be my doctor then?" I asked.

"Yes. I'll take over your treatment if that's what you decide to do," he said.

"Yes! I would love for you to be my doctor!" I said, overjoyed at the news.

I was entering the world of the unknown, but there was one thing that I did know; I would follow Dr. Siegel to the ends of the earth. I trusted him, and even if I didn't make it, I would always know that I was in the best hands possible.

CHAPTER TWENTY-ONE

Children's Hospital

"I've never stayed overnight in a hospital," I said to the nurse who called to talk to me about my upcoming hospital stay.

"Oh, just pack like you are going on vacation. Bring a toothbrush, toothpaste, pajamas, whatever you would normally pack to take on a trip," she replied. Suddenly I got slightly excited. This was my thought process. Vacation - swimming - pool - oooh they have a pool - I wonder if they have yoga classes - Which then led me to ask...

"So, should I bring a bathing suit?"

"No, you will not need a bathing suit," she kindly replied.

That's right, back to reality. I was going to Children's Hospital to get chemotherapy because I had cancer. Although, I still think it would be a great idea to have yoga classes and, yes, even a pool at a hospital. Get your patients active! By the way I actually did ask about yoga on my first day in the hospital. The answer to that question was also, "No." There could have been these incredible classes that were free at the hospital and I would have never known about them unless I asked. Sorry for the digression, back to cancer.

Children's Hospital was not like adult hospitals. It was bright, colorful and didn't have any weird odors like other hospitals. Yes, this is a big one for me. You have to admit that there is a certain medical, sterile odor that you associate with hospitals. It is probably just cleaning products or even medical supplies, but there is a certain smell. Well, I do not like that smell. I do not have good memories of that smell. So, I was overjoyed when I sniffed around and didn't smell a hospital. Excellent!

Everyone was so nice at Children's Hospital. My first nurse, Cami, was the one who checked me in and ended up being my nurse for the majority of my stays. She took her time and answered all of my questions, which I really appreciated. She gave me copies of my blood-work, which I would put into my notebook. Cami knew that I kept all of these papers. I was keeping track of my progress. Nurses and doctors are great, but people make mistakes. If I took an active role in my treatment, then I could help make sure that everything went according to plan. It made me feel like I wasn't at the whim of whatever doctor or nurse was treating me at the moment or whether or not they had all of the information in front of them. I had taken some of the control back and kept a copy of my chemotherapy protocol, my most recent blood work, and my biopsy results. It felt good to not look doe-eyed into a doctor or nurse's eyes, hoping that they had all of the information. It relieved some of my anxiety to have that notebook with me every time I went to the hospital.

Cami answered all of my questions. I found out that there were certain chemotherapies I couldn't get if I had taken another medication within twenty-four hours. Then there was methotrexate, a bright yellow chemotherapy. The important thing to know about methotrexate is that after twenty-four hours you need to take something called a leucovorin rescue. It's just a little pill, but what it does is it stops that particular chemo from damaging your organs. So of course at the twenty-four hour mark I would be watching the clock, and if I didn't have the medication on the dot, then I would call the nurses. Hey, they told me twenty-four hours; I wanted it in twenty-four hours.

Cami took time to explain what everything meant. It felt like she genuinely cared. Sometimes she would just come into my room to talk and keep me company, which I thought was really sweet. It was weird to be there because I was the only adult. Nurses would come in, look at my chart, then look at me, then back at the chart, confused at why a twenty-five year old was in the bed.

The floor that I was being treated on was Four East. It was the floor where kids with cancer were treated. I have to say that when I was first diagnosed with cancer it was easy to feel sorry for myself. Why me? I was only twenty-five. Well, that completely ended for me when I saw those kids. I saw toddlers who were just learning how to walk in the hallways. This one kid had a helmet on and would hold onto his IV with his parent walking beside him as he learned how to walk at the same time as he was getting chemotherapy. He was being treated for cancer just like I was. The difference was that he didn't know any better. He didn't know to be sad or that this wasn't normal. He was just learning how to walk.

The instant I saw these kids of various ages going through exactly what I was going through, or worse, I couldn't feel sorry for myself. I prayed to God to give their cancer, their pain to me so that I could go through it for them. If there had been some way for me to endure all of the pain in the world so that they didn't have to, I would have. Children should not have cancer - period - end of story.

When I got to the hospital they put in a PICC line to give me chemo. A PICC line goes into your arm with a catheter that leads to your heart. This was only temporary; they wanted to give me a port. A port is a device that is implanted under the skin. There is a catheter that goes into your vein, and the port allows easy access for chemotherapy. Instead of trying to find a mangled vein, they just hook your port up, and you are good to go. Some people have ports with tubes that stick out of their chest. Mine was a little different; it was completely under my chest. The only way I can really describe it is if you picture a doorbell. The area outside of where you press the doorbell was anchored to my chest. The area you press was actually a rubber stopper that they could access with a needle. Then there was a catheter that went from that device into my vein. The nurses just had to stick the needle (a one inch needle) into my port to start chemo or draw a blood. It was wonderful!

My port was difficult to access because it was slightly askew. I had some nurses miss on me. They felt so bad. They had not missed in years and then they missed on me. Honestly, it never mattered if they missed because I couldn't feel anything in the area by the incision. This was way better than watching nurses dig around for my veins. Did I mention that the port was wonderful?

When they first told me that I needed to get a port, they said that Dr. Siegel had recommended a double port, instead of a single port. What did that mean? It meant a bigger device with two rubber stoppers to access so that they could give me two different IV's at the same time if they needed to.

"Will I have a bigger scar?" I asked the nurse.

"Yes, it will be a little bit longer," she said.

Well, I didn't want a big scar on my chest. I mean what about that modeling career that I was never going to have? What would my future boyfriend think? Then I had an epiphany... I was fighting for my life. It didn't matter if I had a big scar or a small scar, just as long as I was alive.

"Okay, I want the double port," I said to the nurse. I liked to refer to it as the Cadillac of ports. It made me feel special (it's the little things). With the Cadillac of ports I could get hydration and chemo at the same time if I needed it. If some chemotherapies couldn't go through the same IV, they could always use the second port. *Go big or go home* the saying goes, so I went big.

It felt really weird to have this foreign body in my chest at first. It was uncomfortable to sleep on my side when it was in or to move that arm across my chest when I was putting on my seat belt. Suddenly there was fullness that hadn't been there before, but I got used to it and ended up falling in love with my double port.

I felt safe at Children's Hospital. It was a home away from home. In fact, if I had a choice between home and the hospital I would have rather been at Children's. I knew that if I got sick, they would take care of me. I was in good hands. I was home. I was home with great doctors and nurses and my very own Cadillac of ports!

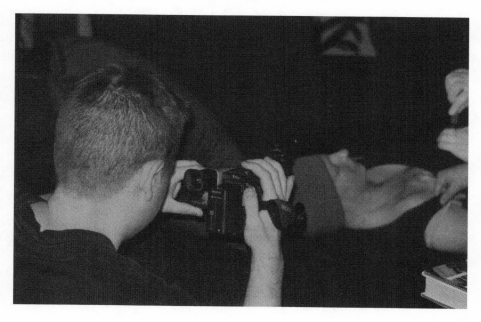

CHAPTER TWENTY-TWO

My Five-Year-Old Roommate

As I walked down the hallway, pushing my IV with one hand, I realized that no one else was around. It was the perfect time to try out what I had seen the kids do. Here and there I would see a kid pushing his IV, then hop onto the bottom of the IV where the wheels were and ride it for a few feet. *Oooh, that looks dangerous*, I thought ...*and like sooo much fun!*

I mean, come on, we were battling cancer, but lets have a little bit of fun. This was my opportunity. No one was around so I didn't have to worry about being a bad example for the kids or the nurses yelling at me. It was the perfect time. I picked up speed as I walked next to the IV pole in my hospital issued socks, then with a giddy smile, jumped onto the bottom. "Wheeeee!"

For a moment I was free. I felt the wind against my face. It was as if I weren't in a hospital and this object that I was riding on wasn't an IV pole. I was transported to a grocery store. Stay with me on this one.

I used to love to do the same thing in the grocery store. You know, take a few quick strides, then jump on to the bottom of a shopping cart and glide with it. That's what it reminded me of, making fun moments out of ordinary ones. In the middle of my blissful moment gliding on my IV pole on the 4th floor of Children's Hospital I got a little nervous. I was hooked up to this thing with tape and needles and tubes. If I fell, it could be very uncomfortable and a bit embarrassing to explain. I put one foot down to slow myself and then hopped off. I was back in the world of Four East, and I was still a cancer patient pushing my IV pole, but I had this magical moment of being free.

One morning I woke up in my hospital bed to the sounds of a new roommate who had moved in. There was a curtain between us so I couldn't see who she was. Since I was being treated at a children's hospital it was normal for me to have younger roommates. I had ones who were ten years old and twelve years old. From the voices I heard from the other side of the curtain it seemed like this was a younger roommate. My eyes felt heavy from being awoken at various times of the night to get my blood pressure taken. I quickly fell back to sleep while my new roommate was getting settled into our room.

Later on my new roommate and her mom passed by my bed and saw that I was awake, "You were sleeping earlier when we came in. Hi, I'm Erika, and this is Bailey."

Bailey was smiling, and shyly looked down and back up, "Hi," she said with the most adorable voice.

She was only five years old and newly diagnosed with leukemia. She had been through a round of chemotherapy at another hospital but then ended up at CHLA. Bailey had already lost her hair, but still had her beautiful brown eyebrows and the best smile around. She looked like a tiny angel. It broke my heart that she had to go through chemotherapy like me.

Erika dropped Bailey off at the playroom then came back and talked to me about her and what they had been through. It seemed like it was always a similar story when it came to leukemia. A child is overly tired or starts bruising very easily for no apparent reason. I've even heard some say their child started favoring a leg because the other one was bothering them. The stories often go that they see their primary care physician who simply says that they are kids and they will get bruises or maybe the child is seeking attention or to give them Tylenol and let them rest. Then after months of not getting better, they either see another doctor or that same doctor takes a blood sample. The blood sample always tells the story. Their white blood cell counts are through the roof, which is extremely bad news. They are told their child has leukemia and before they know it, their lives are turned upside down. I was surprised by how many stories I heard about these kids not being correctly diagnosed when their parents first took them to the doctor.

Maybe an hour later Bailey walked back into the room. Her IV was adorned with pink and purple colored ribbons.

"Oooh! You look like a princess! I want my IV to look like that!" I told her.

She gushed with pride and happiness.

"They decorated it for me," she said in a very shy voice.

"Well, it is just the most beautiful thing I have ever seen!"

"Maybe they can decorate yours."

Then her mom came over and started talking to Bailey.

"Bye!" she said as she walked to her side of the room. It was official. I adored her, and I quickly became a friend of the family. We would see each other again during our other hospital stays and roomed together when it was possible.

Sometimes I would hear her in pain. It was the same pain that I felt, but it was a five-year-old going through it. I would lie in my hospital bed and pray to God to take away her pain and give it to me. *Please, God, give me her pain. Give me her cancer.* There are things in this world that I will never understand, and one of them is why children get cancer.

When I told Bailey stories about being a dolphin trainer, her face would light up. "I want to meet a dolphin," she said in her bashful voice with a smile.

"One day we'll go to SeaWorld, and I'll introduce you to a dolphin, okay?"

"Okay," she said with a huge smile on her face.

I envisioned the whole thing. We would both be healthy with hair on our heads again, and these moments in the hospital and the cancer would be a distant memory. I wanted to get her into a wetsuit so she could see what it was like to be up close with the dolphins. We would have fun and take pictures together, and we would be on the other side of cancer, healthy, happy, and living a dream we had while in the hospital together.

It was a wonderful dream, but we still had a lot of chemotherapy to go through before we would be better, and Bailey's cancer required years of treatment. There was also that whole surviving thing that we needed to accomplish. There was a lot we had to go through in order to live that dream.

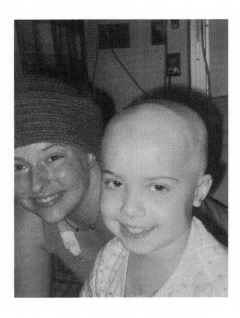

CHAPTER TWENTY-THREE

Blood Work

Blood work rules all. If your white blood cell count is too low, then you can't receive the chemo you need to kill the cancer. You're also more susceptible to infections because you don't have an immune system. The doctors let me know at the beginning of chemo that if I ever got a fever while on treatment, I needed to go to the emergency room. A fever meant my body was trying to fight something off. There would be a rude awakening when my body discovered that there were no white blood cell (WBC) ninjas available to kill the intruder. I was defenseless with a low WBC count.

I knew that if my WBC count was too low, they would not let me return to the hospital to receive the chemotherapy that I needed to kill the cancer. Part of my treatment called for me to give myself shots once a day after I came home from the hospital. It was a drug called Neupogen that helped increase my white blood cell count, which meant I could return to the hospital and get back to killing the cancer.

I had a nurse come to my aunt's house to show me how to give myself an injection. She made it seem relatively easy. First, you get your needle ready. I had to switch out the needle that came with the syringe with a smaller one. Then I needed to draw up the Neupogen. Next was the fun part, grab some skin from your leg and inject the Neupogen.

It all seemed easy enough except I really didn't like injecting myself with Neupogen. It literally would take me a half hour to get up the courage to stick the needle into my leg. I would sit there with the needle hovering above my pinched skin on my thigh, waiting until the right moment to inject myself. The right moment would have been when someone came in and said, "Stop! You don't have to inject yourself anymore!" This mysterious person never came and yelled that though. Eventually I had to go through with the injection.

One of my aunt's friends heard that I was having problems injecting myself. She offered to do it for me since she had experience giving insulin injections to a relative. It sounded like a good enough idea. As long as I didn't have to do it, right? We sat on the couch in the living room where there was plenty of light as we prepared for the injection. She got everything ready and then pinched some skin on my thigh. As I looked at the pinched skin, I noticed that she had her other hand raised really high above her head. I looked up with squinted eyes. *What's that in her hand? Oh My God! It's the needle!* I thought. The needle was in her clenched fist over her head in a crazy, serial killer stabbing motion. Whoa! Whoa! No counting or asking if I'm ready? No warm up to the event? No thirty minutes of hemming and hawing? The sun glistened off the needle as it hung high in the air above me. After my mind processed what was happening, my mouth started to form the word, "WAIT," but before I was able to get the word out the glistening needle left its position in the sun and plummeted into my leg at full velocity. My heart nearly jumped out of my chest.

I thanked her for her help and later told her I would be doing it myself from now on. At least when I took a half an hour to inject myself, I had control. I mean, who raises their hand above their head to give someone an injection? Do you really need that much velocity to get the needle in? And doesn't it decrease your accuracy when it is so far away? Who does that? That was so scary!

CHAPTER TWENTY-FOUR

The Healer

"**M**y friend told me about this healer. Do you want to meet her?" Aunt Susan asked.

"Mmm... okay," I responded.

Aunt Susan's friend raved about this woman who was considered a "healer." I guess it couldn't hurt. It might be interesting. We drove down to her place right outside of L.A. It was a residence. As we pulled into the driveway, I wanted to back out of the whole thing. This just seemed too weird, but we were there and had driven a long way so here we go.

The healer had me lie down on a table and hovered her hands above different parts of my body. She told me what parts were stressed and then put stickers with a hand written number on those parts. She wanted me to keep those stickers there for a few days.

What she didn't know was that I spent most of my free time in the warm waters of a bathtub. Those stickers didn't stand a chance. A nice warm bath was the only thing that made me feel better. I would spend hours soaking in the tub. Sometimes (I know this is really bad) I would even take naps in the bathtub. I would make sure the water was really low so I wouldn't drown. Then I would curl up and go to sleep. I can't believe I'm admitting this to you.

Of course when I got home from the healer, I had to take a bath. Not only did I take naps in the bathtub when I felt really bad, but I also read and did some great thinking. It was almost a hobby, but I can't write that down when I am asked about my hobbies because I would simply be misunderstood. All I'm saying is that I am a bath addict.

When I got home from the healer with all of my stickers over the parts that needed extra healing, I couldn't avoid the bathtub. There was a moment when I thought about not taking a bath. Then that moment passed, and before I knew it, I was splashing around in the warm, comforting water. I thought maybe the stickers would stay on; I just wouldn't scrub. Well, they didn't, and before I knew it, I had all of these numbered stickers floating next to me in the tub. Whoops.

There was one thing from the healer that I really liked and practiced daily. She told me to say, "I'm cancer free" seven times in a row each day. I took this to the next level. I said it hundreds of times, but would count them by sevens. I said this an enormous amount of times when I was scared or when I was getting my scans (which can be scary when you know that the scans are looking for cancer). It felt good to say those words.

I'm cancer free. I'm cancer free. I'm cancer free. I'm cancer free. I'm cancer free. I'm cancer free. I'm cancer free.

I'm cancer free. I'm cancer free. I'm cancer free. I'm cancer free. I'm cancer free. I'm cancer free. I'm cancer free.

I'm cancer free. I'm cancer free. I'm cancer free. I'm cancer free. I'm cancer free. I'm cancer free. I'm cancer free.

I'm cancer free. I'm cancer free. I'm cancer free. I'm cancer free. I'm cancer free. I'm cancer free. I'm cancer free.

I'm cancer free. I'm cancer free. I'm cancer free. I'm cancer free. I'm cancer free. I'm cancer free. I'm cancer free.

I'm cancer free. I'm cancer free. I'm cancer free. I'm cancer free. I'm cancer free. I'm cancer free. I'm cancer free.

I'm cancer free. I'm cancer free. I'm cancer free. I'm cancer free. I'm cancer free. I'm cancer free. I'm cancer free.

CHAPTER TWENTY-FIVE

Cookies

My aunt's ex-husband and his friends got together and baked some cookies with a little something special in it for me. Wasn't that sweet? It was probably the only time he had ever cooked. In the freezer there was a bag containing the cookies with a label that said, "Do Not Touch!" My aunt offered me the cookies, but I didn't take her up on it immediately. One day I decided to try one. The "special ingredient" was supposed to help with appetite, and I had lost mine so I ate a cookie. I didn't really feel anything and decided to take a nap (in a bed, not a bathtub). When I woke up, I was hungry and feeling really weird. I was on the second floor and needed to make it to the first floor for some food. Wow, it took everything in me to get down those stairs. All I could see were dark swirly colors, like a big nebula in space, in front of me. I could barely see the stairs. It must have taken me an hour to get down to the first floor. Was I tripping? Precisely what did they add to these cookies? When I finally made it to the last step, I vowed to never leave the first floor again.

I made my way to the kitchen, which was a whole lot easier than the stairs. My uncle had bought me some Wetzel's pretzels. I loved them, especially with mustard. I got out my pretzel and a bottle of mustard. It was a typical yellow, roundish plastic container of mustard. I sat at the table and got ready to enjoy this feast. As I grabbed the mustard container and brought it up to the pretzel to put a little on the bite I was about to eat, I noticed something strange. The mustard bottle had a tail. I looked at it again and not only did it have a tail, but it also had ears. Yet, it was still a mustard bottle. It just had a tail and ears. What the heck did they put in that cookie? Was I seriously tripping? *Okay, this is not a mouse. It is just my imagination,* I told myself. I shook the mustard bottle and got rid of the ears, but the tail was still there. I ate the pretzel with the mustard but had to keep telling myself it was just my mind playing tricks on me. It was the strangest thing ever. The next day I thanked my aunt for the cookies, but told her I wouldn't be having anymore.

CHAPTER TWENTY-SIX

Hospitalized

One day I was feeling very weak. I called Dr. Siegel and told him I wasn't expecting to feel as bad as I did. He asked me to go to the mirror and pull down my lower eyelid.

"Is it red or white?" he asked.

"It's a really light pink, almost a white color."

"Okay, you are probably just low on your red blood cells. We'll have you come in tomorrow to get a blood transfusion. Now, if you get a fever before that, you should come in immediately."

That night Kevin, Brian, and I watched TV downstairs. Kevin moved into my aunt's house to help me while I was going through my treatment. Brian was between jobs and decided to fly out to be by my side. It was great having the two of them there with me. When I was tired, I could just listen to them talk to each other and not be worried about entertaining them.

I got up from the couch to go to bed, but I was so weak from the chemo and low blood counts that I blacked out every-time I stood up. Everything just turned black, but I didn't pass out. I could hear everything just fine. No one knew that I couldn't see. I would just breathe through it, then my vision would slowly come back, and I could start to walk.

When I walked, my legs would buckle from underneath me because I was so weak.

"I want to go upstairs to bed, but I'm not looking forward to the stairs," I told Kevin and Brian as I stood in the same place for a little too long.

"I'll give you a ride," Brian offered.

"Oh, no, I'm okay. Thanks."

Before I knew it Brian had picked me up and was carrying me up the stairs.

"Thank you, Brian."

I went to bed that night feeling awful. It was hard to sleep. My throat was really hurting me from the mucositis, which made it difficult to sleep. Then I started to notice that I was sweating. This might be a good time to get out of bed and find a thermometer. Ugh, getting out of bed. Okay, here we go. Stand up - black out- breathe - don't move - vision is coming back - time to walk. I was sure that I was just being paranoid, but I should be safe and take it anyway. Sure enough, I had a fever. Now Dr. Siegel's words echoed in my mind. I had actually heard it a number of times from nurses and other doctors. They say it in a nonchalant way, but they were always very serious about getting the message out. It's almost a little mantra that they have. "If you get a fever and have a low WBC, you need to go to the hospital. Don't worry about making an appointment or calling your doctor. Just go to the hospital."

At 1:00 a.m. I called Kevin on his cell phone.

"Guess who has a fever?" I asked Kevin.

"Oh, no, really?" Kevin asked.

"Yup," I replied.

"Alright, I'll let Brian know."

Kevin pulled up his car, and Brian helped me carry my overnight bag. We drove down to the hospital and arrived in record time.

After waiting at the emergency room for a bit and Kevin filming me for eight seconds on the bench, a doctor arrived to check on me. He asked a few questions which I painfully answered. Then he put me in a wheelchair and brought me to my room on the fourth floor. Ahhh, I was home. I was safe. They could help me. They got a blood sample as soon as I was upstairs and then hooked me up to an IV with antibiotics. When my blood work came back, it showed that my WBC was .1. The normal range is 4.50-11.00. I was .1, which was not good. The chemo was doing a number on my blood counts. Next they showed me my hemoglobin (HGB) was 7.0. Normal range is 12.0 to 15.5. That explained why I was so weak and light headed.

Because my hemoglobin was so low, they needed to give me a blood transfusion. I had never had one before and wasn't excited about my first one. It made the whole situation feel a lot more serious. They hooked up my port to a bag of blood and before I knew it, the blood was flowing into my veins. I just turned over and slept for the first few hours that I received the transfusion. When I woke up, I had some energy and color had returned to my face. Soon my nurse came in and took down the empty bag of blood on my IV and replaced it with a new one. All in all I had about three blood transfusions during my hospital stay.

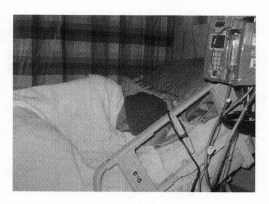

While all of this was happening, Kevin and Brian were giving me time to rest. They found the family waiting room, which had a bunch of chairs connected to each other in a long line and a TV. Kevin and Brian were the only ones in there so they decided to "redecorate" the room. They moved the long line of connected chairs together so they could put up their feet. After all they hadn't slept yet, and at that point it was early morning. Then they decided to turn the camera on themselves. Kevin narrated from behind the camera as he filmed Brian with his feet up on the chairs.

"It's really late or no... it's really early. It's 4:30, no, it's almost 5:00 now.... Brian and I are in the waiting room, Joy is in her room now, hopefully sleeping, probably not because she is in a lot of pain. Anyway we have decided to make the living room/ waiting room a little more comfortable. We've ripped the seats off the wall so that we can use them as foot rests. Anyway, the things we do for you Joy! We love you."

People started arriving steadily throughout the day to visit me. Aunt Susan had made some phone calls and told people that they needed to come see me that day... just in case. People were coming in to say goodbye, but I was feeling better. The blood transfusion made me feel like a million bucks. It hit home again that surviving this experience was not a sure thing.

Some people came in and looked at me with sadness in their eyes and embraced me. Others hung out and watched movies. At one point when it was just Kevin and Brian in my room, I asked them to play charades. I love charades. There was one strange hitch though. I was tired and didn't have the energy to play... I just wanted them to play. They started, and I closed my eyes.

One of them said, "You aren't even going to watch?"

"No, I want to listen," I said with a smile, realizing how ridiculous it was, but not caring.

So I listened as one begrudgingly acted out a clue and the other guessed. The best part was that with my eyes closed, I made one guess and I got it!

"Titanic!" I said with my eyes closed.

"That's it!" Brian said.

"What? How did you get that?" Kevin asked.

"I really like charades," I answered.

I lay in bed with my eyes closed and a big smile on my face, giggling to myself whenever I thought about it.

As the day wore on people started to leave, and by evening I was by myself, which was just fine. I enjoyed my alone time. It also meant that I could be naked. No, not completely naked, just my head. I could take off my blue cap that I wore religiously and give my noggin' some breathing space. I sat there in my dark room watching TV while rubbing my hand over my baldhead.

My bed was next to a door with three large diamond shaped windows in a vertical line. As I rested in my hospital bed with my baldhead exposed, I saw the light from the windows in my door get obstructed. Some woman was frantically looking inside. She was obviously looking for someone, and I was positive that someone was not me. I thought she would leave at any moment. Then the door opened.

Are you kidding me? You have the wrong room, I thought.

The woman stood in front of me for a moment, silhouetted by the hallway light in my dark room.

"Joy... ?" the woman asked. I recognized the voice.

"Mom?"

She walked closer, and I could see her. My mom had come to be with me.

"Oh my gosh, Mom! I can't believe you're here! You flew out from Hawaii?"

"Aunt Susan said you weren't doing well, so I grabbed the first flight out," she said.

I was overcome with emotion. My mom had come to say goodbye to me. She did the hardest thing imaginable for a mother and stayed away until she simply couldn't anymore. Then she ignored her stupid daughter and flew out to be by her side. I did need her, and I was so happy to see her.

"I brought you a tuberose flower lei. I know they're your favorite," she said as she smiled and pulled a flower lei out of a plastic bag and placed it around my neck.

The fragrance brought back wonderful memories of Hawaii. Unfortunately, because my immune system was non-existent, I wasn't allowed to have flowers. I took a few last illegal sniffs of the tuberose before walking the lei over to the nurses' station for them to enjoy.

My mom was there. She wasn't going anywhere, and I was happy to have her. All of the things I was worried about didn't happen. I didn't have to be strong for her; she was strong for me. She didn't distract the doctors. She was there to love me and help take care of me. She even found ways to make me dinner while I was in the hospital. It was so nice.

A couple of days after I was hospitalized, the nurses gave me some liquid medication to help me poop. So here is the long and short of it. I got incredibly constipated while going through chemotherapy, which was made worse by my overnight stays in the hospital. The chemotherapy already can cause constipation, but then I would get stage fright when I had to poop (I can't believe I'm telling you about this). In the hospital there were two people to a room, plus there was an IV pole to tote around. The IV pole didn't fit in the bathroom so the door was always a little ajar in order for the IV pole to be outside while the IV tubing prevented the door from closing. To top all of this off you had to poop and pee into something called a hat. The hat is the name for what is supposed to be put in the toilet before you poop or pee so that they can collect and measure it. Yeah, I could not do that. Could not. Absolutely no chance in heck that I was going to be able to poop into a "hat." It got to a point where I would sneak off to the public restroom on the floor and try to poop in privacy. Then I had plenty of time. I didn't have to worry about my roommate needing to use the restroom or the visitors in the room listening to me. The nurses eventually caught onto this. When I explained my situation, they told me to tell them what it looked like and I was off the hook for the "hat."

They gave me Colace pills to help with the constipation. They did not work for me in any way, shape, or form. When my mom was there, they wanted to try something new, mineral oil. The only problem was that I really, really, (more than you will ever know) hate liquid medication of any kind. It has always taken me about a half an hour or more to take liquid NyQuil (the green kind especially). My stepmom would line up other things for me to take after I got up the courage to swallow the disgusting, and I mean DISGUSTING, green medicine. The first was water, then apple juice, then coffee ice cream, and then I was okay.

The nurse came in with a few tablespoons of mineral oil in a cup. I was hesitant. My mom was there with me when I told the nurse about my concern, but the nurse wanted me to try it anyway. The worst thing that could happen was my hard poop would rip a hole in me, and then I would have poop in an open wound, which would have been a bad situation with no immune system. It was more important for them to get me to drink the mineral oil than to worry about whether or not I hated liquid medication. After some deliberation and huffing and puffing, I took it. Then I waited for the world to end immediately afterward, but to my surprise I was fine. Great! I took it without a problem! I sat there and talked to my mom for about five minutes. Then without warning it came right back up. My body said, "Thanks, but no thanks. Return to sender." I went from mid-conversation with Mom to having eyes as big as saucers and a mouthful of mineral oil and vomit. I couldn't make it to the bathroom. I was hooked up to IVs and heart monitors. It wasn't going to happen in time. I looked at my mom and signaled for her to get me something. I was thinking trashcan. A trashcan would be a good size. It made sense to me. She ran around the room for a few moments, frantically looking for something. Finally she came back. Sweet relief! I have something to throw up in. She quickly threw me a small, shallow, rectangular tissue box and looked at me like, "Go ahead. You can vomit now." She had gotten me a tissue box... I looked at the tissue box, then back at her like she was crazy, with my cheeks out like a blowfish. I made a guttural sound and pointed to the garbage can. She understood what I wanted and quickly grabbled the garbage can and gave it to me. Ahhh.

We laughed about that for a while afterward. I still think it's funny that she ran around and came back with a small tissue box. Sometimes the best moments come at the worst times.

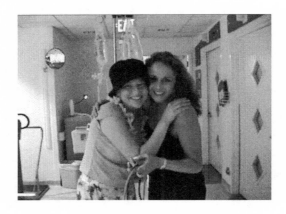

CHAPTER TWENTY-SEVEN

Valentine's Day

"Len, you have prayed for me a lot over the years. Now you know what you have to do when you get to Heaven... you need to pray for Joy."

That was what Aunt Susan said to Grandpa Len as he lay in the retirement home about to die. The nurses called in a priest to give him his last rites. He had outlived his wife and all of his friends. It was time for him to go back to Heaven. I believe that we all came from Heaven, and when we are done here on earth, we will return to Heaven.

Aunt Susan returned home after seeing Grandpa Len and told me what she had said to him. It was nice knowing that people had me in their prayers, and the ultimate, of course, was for Grandpa Len to pray for me in Heaven... a former Catholic priest praying for me in Heaven? That has got to count a little more. I know this may sound weird, but I never prayed for myself to be well. I talked to God, but I never prayed or begged to get better. I didn't bargain. I figured that this was something that I would learn from. I would learn a lesson from my cancer, whether I lived or died.

My dad explained death to me when I was little, and I still like what he said. He told me that people are here for as much time as they need. Sometimes we just need to be here on earth for a few minutes, sometimes an entire lifetime. We are here to learn lessons and to help teach others lessons too.

So when I found out I had cancer, I thought it was a lesson I was here to learn. At least that was a nice way of looking at it. There was a purpose to my cancer, whether it taught others a lesson or the lesson was for me. God thought I was strong enough to handle this or else he wouldn't have given it to me. That is how I looked at it. I was never mad at him or had to forgive him.

When I was about ten, I REALLY wanted to visit my best friend Jen. I prayed to God to see her. It was a test.

"Okay, God, if You really are out there and I pray to see my best friend, then if I get to see her, You exist."

Well, I didn't see her, and I realized how stupid that was, but I have never prayed for anything that I have really wanted since then. I have been afraid that the opposite will happen. I have merely hoped for one thing or another and thanked God for what I have in my life.

Still, having someone that had been a member of the church pray for me would be pretty cool. Grandpa Len would look over me when he reached Heaven and pray for me. It was a nice image. My tall Irish angel, who enjoyed playing golf and telling jokes. Things have got to turn out well with a super cool angel like that. It meant a lot that Aunt Susan whispered that to him.

The next day my aunt received a phone call from the home. My aunt looked shocked as she got off the phone. "They said they have never seen anything like it. He is up and talking. He is joking around with the nurses like nothing happened," she said.

"But, I thought he was about to pass?" I asked.

"He was... I got there right after they had given him his last rites." Then she smiled and said, "You know what? I'll bet you anything that he is hanging on until he knows that you are okay."

It was a nice thought.

Months passed, and he was still hanging on. I went to visit him with Aunt Susan. He didn't recognize me. I was bald at the time and wearing an auburn wig, but I still assumed that he would recognize me. He didn't, but he did talk to the stranger in the room about me.

"Hi, Grandpa. Do you like my new hairstyle?" I asked him. He looked at me, but he didn't see me.

"There is this beautiful girl in San Diego. She's just beautiful! Do you know that she plays with those dolphins down there in San Diego, and can you believe it, they told her she has cancer? Lymphoma. What a shame," he said as he shook his head with a look of sadness.

"It's me, Grandpa," I said. He looked at me, but he was looking at a stranger. He didn't know that same girl he spoke about was standing before him. I thought about taking off my wig and saying, "Look, Grandpa, it's me. I'm bald like you," but, that could backfire. I didn't want to confuse him or make him upset.

After a few moments of this, I could feel the tears start to well up. I gave him a hug goodbye, and turned around to leave. I was about to lose it. I simply turned around and looked at him one last time with a red face and tears, "Goodbye," I said as I waved to him and smiled through tears. He didn't know me. I'm sure he had no idea why the stranger in the room had tears streaming down her face as she said goodbye.

Three days after my ER trip in the middle of the night, I was on my way home to Ventura. I was very aware that my story may not end in survival, and I wanted to be at peace if that time came. I decided to thank God for everything. I got out my video camera. It was the only way I could get out all of my thoughts... the good and the scary.

"I just wanted to thank God if I survive, and I also want to thank God if I go out of remission and die. I know that there are lessons that I need to learn, and I will learn great things from them. So, thank you," I said to my video camera.

On Valentine's Day Dr. Siegel ordered scans to see what was happening with the cancer. This would determine my future. The whole time that the scans were being done, I repeated the words, "I'm cancer free," over and over again. I probably said it over a thousand times as my body was scanned for evidence of cancer. Then I had to wait a few hours to hear the results from Dr. Siegel. The hours ticked by, and finally it was time. Brian and Kevin were in the room with me when Dr. Siegel came in. I prepared for the worst. *It will be okay. I'm strong. I can do this,* I thought. Dr Siegel then started to talk.

"The scans show that there is…" The blood started to drain from my face. "… no evidence of cancer in your body," he said.

"Nothing? The stuff that was around my lungs and behind my heart?" I asked.

"It's gone. You are cancer free. Now you still have two more rounds of chemotherapy that you have to complete, but this is very good news," he said with a smile.

When I got out of the hospital, I turned on my phone to let everyone know the good news. I saw that I had a message from Aunt Susan. "I'm sorry, Honey, but I want you to know that Grandpa Len passed away this morning. I love you," she said in the message.

What? Oh my gosh! He really did hang on until he knew I was okay, I thought. Aunt Susan had told him to pray for me and he did. I imagined God talking to him, "It's okay, Len. She's okay. You can come home now."

I called Aunt Susan crying.

"The cancer is gone. The scans show no cancer. What time did he pass?" I asked.

"Oh, Joy, that is the best news! Len passed around 11:00 this morning, Honey," she said.

"My scans were at 10:00 a.m. He knew I was okay!" I said.

I'm sure Aunt Susan had simply said he was holding on until he knew I was okay as a nice sentiment, a nice reason for him to not pass away that night. Then it actually happened. He died the same day I found out the cancer was gone. It was more than a coincidence. For the rest of the day when I told people I was cancer free, I also told them about Grandpa Len and how he held on until he knew I was okay. I was a complete mess.

This all happened on Valentine's Day. I found out that I was cancer free, and my grandpa died. When we got back to the house, Brian and Kevin told me they wanted to take me out to dinner for Valentine's Day. They gave me an hour to get ready. I took the opportunity to relax for fifty minutes then get ready, so I was a little late. When I made it downstairs, I walked outside with them, ready to get into Kevin's car. As we left the house, I saw a white stretch limo outside of Aunt Susan's house. I thought it was weird that there was a limo there, and I was a bit annoyed. *Why do they have to block our driveway?* I thought. I started to walk around the limo until I saw them walk toward the limo door.

"We decided to go all out," Brian said.

"Yeah, we thought you could use a little pampering, and now we get to celebrate the good news," Kevin said. I was in shock. When I got into the limo, there was a bouquet of red roses on the seat... for me. I felt like I was in a movie. It was magical.

We had dinner in Santa Barbara, among the living, and celebrated the fantastic news. Then we played miniature golf. It seemed fitting that we played miniature golf on the day that my grandpa died since he had loved golf so much during his lifetime.

Brian eventually flew back home and Kevin stayed with me until I finished my treatment. I had my own team of people making sure I survived. I felt like the luckiest person in the world.

"Thank you, God, for these wonderful friends and for being cancer free. I love you, Grandpa."

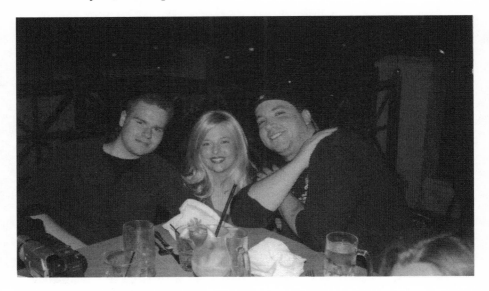

CHAPTER TWENTY-EIGHT

Normal Life

"Now, just go back to normal life." This is what doctors say after you finish your treatment. I had finished my last two rounds of chemotherapy. Going back to normal life seemed amazing, but the problem was I didn't feel normal. I had just fought for my life. I was bald, weak, and suffering from a bit of Post Traumatic Stress Disorder. I didn't know the last part for a while though. I had just spent the last six months fighting for my life, and now I was supposed to be "normal." The doctors brought me to the brink of death and back. Now, just go back to normal life? It just seems like there should be some sort of transition. Maybe a ticker tape parade for such a battle would be an adequate transition, something to mark that I was anything but normal. I was extraordinary! I was a cancer survivor!

No ticker tape parade happened, but I did lock myself up in my room for days and weeks. I was waiting for my hair to grow back before I re-entered normal life. This was probably not a good idea. I totally isolated myself so that I could heal, grow back my hair, and go back to normal... at least that is how I justified it. You might ask how I could stay in my room for days and weeks. Well, there was a restroom attached to the bedroom and people brought me food. I really didn't have to EVER leave if I didn't want to. When someone brought me food, I wouldn't even open the door all the way. A hand would emerge from the room with the door only open about six inches. The mysterious hand would grab the plate from the kind friend or relative, then carefully bring it back through the six inch gap, while leaving it open just long enough to give them my old plates. This is not the picture of "normal life" that doctors envision. What can I say? I'm unique.

I eventually emerged from my hibernation and decided to take water aerobics. My muscles had atrophied from months of bed rest, bathtub marathons, and general inactivity. Water aerobics seemed perfect. Low impact exercise in water seemed like a match made in Heaven for me. On my first day I quickly realized I was the youngest person there by a good thirty years. The other ladies put on swim caps to protect their hair. I simply took my wig off and was ready to go.

The older water aerobics group took me in. Some of them had also battled cancer during their lifetimes. There was even a woman in the class who needed oxygen. There was a long tube that led from her to an oxygen tank on the side of the pool. My imagination went into overdrive during every class. I was sure that I would be the one to trip over the clear plastic tube that floated in the water and accidentally rip it from her nostrils. Then the older ladies would turn on me. My heightened awareness paid off. I safely maneuvered class with no incidents. I was an honorary old lady, and I loved it! It was a nice transition to being normal. I slowly re-entered life.

My hair grew back slowly. At first it was just peach fuzz that required the right light to really see. It felt good to know that something was growing in, but it was so fuzzy. I remembered my great Aunt Anna telling me that if you shave your hair, it will grow back thicker and darker (she was talking about arm hair). Well, I didn't have anything to lose. I mean it was just peach fuzz so one day I decided to shave my head. I lathered up my fuzzy head, got out my Lady Gillette, and shaved my head. It was actually pretty exciting because I was shaving off hair, actual hair that I hadn't had in about six months. It made me realize that I really did have a decent amount of hair. I emerged as a young female Yul Brynner. I had to wait even longer for my hair to grow back. Still I was taking control, and that felt good. About three weeks later I had enough hair to go out into public. It looked like a crew cut. As it grew back it actually looked really cool. I looked like a movie star from the forties with a short wavy hairstyle.

I had to return to the hospital every month to have checkups with Dr. Siegel. If things were good, then he would approve for me to be seen every three months, then every six, and finally I would only have to come in once a year.

During one of my checkups I found out that Bailey was in the hospital getting another round of chemotherapy. Of course I had to visit her! After getting a bill of good health from Dr. Siegel, I went back to Four East to see Bailey. When I walked into the room, she noticed one big change in my appearance. I had hair! She had seen me wear a wig once before, but this time it was actually my real hair. I saw her looking at my new, short, wavy, dark locks. I knew she was thinking it wasn't real, so I said, "It isn't a wig. This is my real hair."

I pulled on my own hair to show that it was attached to my head. She looked skeptical. "Here, you can pull on it to see that it's real." I leaned my head down to her level while she was sitting in the hospital bed. "Go ahead. It's okay." She grabbed a tuft of my hair and yanked just enough to know it wasn't a wig. As I withdrew my hair from her grasp, I saw her face light up and her eyes fill with a vision of the future.

"Oh my gosh! It really is your hair!" she said with a big smile.

"See, this is what your hair will look like when it grows back." At that moment my short, wavy, brown hair was a form of hope for her. She saw me when I was sick and bald and fighting for my life, and now I looked normal. The hair on my head represented hope that one day she would be on the other side of cancer too.

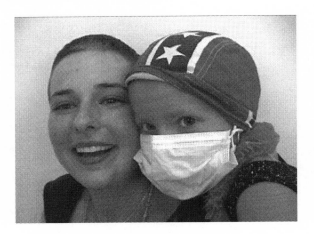

CHAPTER TWENTY-NINE

Lost

I would like to say that after cancer I bounced back and everything was perfect. Little bluebirds landed on my shoulder and adorable cartoon mice made my bed. But, it was not perfect. I was lost. My path in life had been derailed, and I was trying to forge another path with a machete through thick brush. I couldn't see where I was going, just what was immediately in front of me.

My stepmom would say, "You are exactly where you are supposed to be," but I just felt so lost and not anywhere close to being on the right path. I've always wanted to find my purpose in life. "Who am I? Why am I here?" This was my first memory from a crib in my mom's house. Now my first memory was haunting me. I wanted to get to my purpose and get back to my life's journey.

CHAPTER THIRTY

Wrong Turn

As an official member of the "normal life club" I decided to accept an invitation to a Fourth of July party. A friend of mine from film school invited me to a small gathering at her house for the Fourth. Social outings before were strictly prohibited because of my low white blood cell counts. Before I couldn't be around anyone who was sick because my body couldn't protect itself, but that wasn't the case anymore. I was done with my treatment and my counts were almost back to normal. I could actually accept this offer. Now there was the matter of me looking a little different. At this point my hair was long enough to not wear a wig, but it looked like I just joined the army the day prior and had my head buzzed. Still it was enough hair for me to not wear my itchy, hot wigs. Don't get me wrong. They are fun, but it's nice to be able to just go naked. (Without a wig is the naked I'm talking about!)

When I got to the party, it was a small group of very close friends. They had obviously been briefed on my story because they were full of questions about the cancer, chemotherapy, blood transfusions, and my port (you know the "Cadillac of ports" that I had surgically placed in my chest). It was always fun showing off my port because you could see a lump and feel a solid object under my skin. I was used to it and had fallen in love with my port. It saved my veins and was a source of security for me. I didn't care if people thought it was weird. It helped me receive the chemotherapy and blood transfusions that saved my life.

I met a guy named Dave at the party. Dave and I hit it off. We bantered back and forth. I was determined not to seem sick or fragile. It was easy to be myself around him. Actually, I was pretty sure he was gay - perfect! Well, he wasn't gay (darn it), and as our friendship grew, he told me he wanted to be more than friends. I told him it was too early for me. I needed to concentrate on healing. He then said that he couldn't be just friends with me and wouldn't be able to be around me without something more. So what did the girl who just stood up to cancer do? She caved. I wanted that friendship. I wanted that normal feeling. I decided to say, "Yes," to a relationship. Plus, let's face it. It's more than slightly flattering that someone who meets you when you have virtually no hair finds you fun, funny, and attractive.

Although I initially did not want to start dating him when I was still getting back on my feet, I found myself in love with the idea that he "fell in love" with me when I had no hair. This started to develop into a great story to tell people and, goodness knows, I am a sucker for a good story even if I am forcing a square peg into a round hole. This... would be... my... fairytale... (it's exhausting trying to make something fit when it really doesn't... I am quite determined though).

CHAPTER THIRTY-ONE

Fairytale?

Girl survives cancer, meets Prince Charming, who ignores the other maidens with gorgeous hair and goes for the girl who has just survived a battle with a horrible monster. He has never seen her true outward beauty, but falls in love with her inward beauty. Girl heals from the battle and turns into a beautiful princess. It sounded awesome! I just couldn't let go of how wonderful it sounded when I said, "He fell in love with me when I was bald."

I spent my time with him and waited to finish this great fairytale. I was in the middle of putting together a documentary on my battle with cancer, and this seemed like a great ending. That was part of my problem. I was trying to write my happy ending before it actually happened.

Dave and I went through ups and downs. Sometimes things were great. Then we would break up because of something stupid. Then he would be on my doorstep, and we would get back together. I can't even remember how many times we broke up over the years we were together. It was that often.

"I've decided to go to law school in Hawaii," Dave said to me one day over dinner.

"Okay, when did you decide this?" I asked with a cocked head and squinted eyes, confused.

"I've been thinking about it for a while, and I wanted to see if you would accompany me?" he said.

"Accompany you?" I asked, wondering if he was saying what I thought he was saying. I think of accompany as being more of a short-term thing... like to the opera.

"Ms. Clausen, I want to know if you will move to Hawaii with me?"

"Oh, wow!" I said. Then I thought about how much I loved Hawaii and how wonderful it was when I lived there during college. It was magical. My life was not going anywhere. I was working in a restaurant while editing my documentary at home, and I felt like a failure. My path in life had been mucked up, and I certainly wasn't where I wanted to be.

"Okay. Yes, I'll move to Hawaii with you," I said.

I sold everything I owned except for my clothes, jewelry, and car. I shipped these things to Hawaii and eagerly waited to shake things up and start a new life. I was on my way to Hawaii and fighting for my fairy tale ending....

CHAPTER THIRTY-TWO

Hawaii, Not Exactly Paradise

"Two Mai Tais," I said to the bartender. He barely made eye contact with me or spoke to me. I watched as he poured the Mai Tai mix and two different types of rum into two glasses. I picked them up, put them on my round server's tray, then carried the drinks over to a small bar table.

"Here you go, two Mai Tais. Would you like to look at a menu?" I asked.

"Not right now," the man said.

As I walked away, my head started to fill with other things. *How did I get here? I was working at my dream job, and now I am HERE serving drinks? I survived CANCER for this? I thought I was meant for more. I thought I was meant for something bigger than this.*

"Joy, it's slow. We are going to cut the second cocktail tonight. You can get out of here," my boss said to me.

I walked back home in my uniform, a dark blue shirt with white shorts that smelled like a restaurant. I was in Waikiki, walking on the main street, Kalakaua Avenue. I put my headphones on and listened to the soundtrack to *Elizabethtown*. There was one scene that I loved in that movie. Orlando Bloom's character was incredibly depressed after a massive failure in his life. Then he started talking to this girl on the phone, and the song "Come Pick Me Up" by Ryan Adams comes on. You can see his demeanor change. You see a spark in him reignite. This song started to play on my ipod. I loved the first line, "When they call your name, will you walk right up with a smile on your face?" I thought about Heaven when I heard this line. Will I walk right up to the gates of heaven with a smile on my face, knowing I did everything I could to fulfill my purpose?

I walked by incredibly expensive stores that I could never afford to buy anything in and people on vacation living their best lives.

Then I started to escape my reality. As Ryan Adams belted out, "Come Pick Me Up" I imagined that I was dancing with my arms stretched out while these people walked by me. I imagined that I was happy and somewhere different from where I was. The light post I walked by turned into a prop that I could grab onto and spin around with one arm out feeling alive. Of course, I wasn't doing that, but my mind was setting me free for brief moments of happiness. Music was bringing me peace when I was deeply depressed with where I was in life. It was a nice break from reality. FADE TO BLACK.

My phone rang and woke me up. I was in my 200 square foot apartment that I shared with Dave. I wanted to get up, but he had his arm and leg over me. *Ahhh!* I felt so suffocated!

I rolled off the bed and fell to the ground to get away, then walked to the bathroom. "Hello!" I said, in an upbeat voice. It was my stepmom, whom I liked to call, Pacific Mommy Fish, a name we coined on a trip to Hawaii when I was little. She would call me her Pacific Baby Fish.

"How are you doing, Pacific Baby Fish?" she asked.

I closed the door, then stepped into the bathtub, and closed the shower curtain... you know, for extra privacy.

"I'm good," I said as I settled into the bathtub, checking to make sure the curtain was closed all the way.

The truth was that I wasn't good. I was in the wrong relationship, in the wrong job. Basically, I was living the wrong life.

Things between Dave and me were not great. He had a tendency to pick on little things that I did or said, even how I walked. It was hard to feel good around someone who was always making comments about what I was doing wrong. In addition, our living situation was less than ideal, but full of interesting facts.

FACT: Dave and I lived in a building that was featured on "Dog the Bounty Hunter" as a hotspot for drug dealers and prostitutes. Of course we didn't know that before we signed the lease.

FACT: The room that we shared was about 200 square-feet. It was supposed to be nicer than other rooms because it had a kitchen. What I didn't realize was that the "kitchen" was inside the bathroom.

"How is that legal?" you may ask. I do not know.

"How is that physically possible?" you may ask.

Well, there was a stainless steel kitchen sink inside the bathroom instead of a bathroom sink, and below the sink there were cabinets with kitchen utensils and *voila*, the owners could say there is a kitchen. Please, never lose the image that the toilet was a couple of feet away and the bathtub even closer. I would literally be using the bathroom when Dave would try to come in because he was hungry. It was just wrong in every way.

FACT: There were always fun surprises in the elevator like an abandoned shopping cart, or moving boxes with no mover, full trash bags, a chair. It kept life interesting. *I wonder what will be in the elevator today?* I would think while waiting for my elevator surprise to arrive. I didn't have much to look forward to, but this kept my life interesting.

I survived cancer for this? This was my fairytale? I didn't get it. I was supposed to do something great with my life. That is why I survived... right? Yet I was sharing an elevator with drug dealers and prostitutes who were going to be busted on future episodes of "Dog the Bounty Hunter." I was working in a restaurant and in a relationship with someone who really didn't make me happy. There had to be something more than this, but when I was in the muck of things, it was hard to see that better days would come. I just had to keep pushing on until the better days were there, even if it was through tears and depression.

"Okay, tell me all about it," my stepmom said.

"Hmm, life is not going the way I expected it to. I'm incredibly depressed, and I have no idea how to write a script for a short movie," I said to her as my voice started to break, and tears streamed down my face.

I had met a great guy named Lloyd Phillips. He was a Hollywood producer at Sony who saw my documentary and believed in me. He recommended I write a great short story, shoot it, and send it to festivals as a way to go right into being a director, but I just couldn't write a story to save my life.

"Joy, this is all part of the journey. You are exactly where you are supposed to be," my stepmom said as tears streamed down my face. I looked up to where I imagined Heaven to be.

"Mom, I'm sitting in an empty bathtub in my clothes with the curtain closed for privacy," I said.

"You know what story I want to see? A story of someone crying in a bathtub with her clothes on. Write that story," she said.

There was a beep on the phone. It was Lloyd calling from California to check on me.

"Mom, I've got to go. It's Lloyd," I said.

"Okay, call me back."

I sat up straight in the bathtub, wiped away my tears, smiled, and took a deep breath, then clicked over.

"Lloyd!" I said in my best "I'm not depressed" voice.

"Hey, how is it over there in Paradise?" he asked.

"Oh, it's beautiful over here. You know, it's Paradise." I replied from my bathroom/kitchen/personal Hell. I could not tell him that things were not great and that I was not happy and that I had fallen on my face after surviving cancer. This was not the way it was supposed to be. I was supposed to flourish. I should be the butterfly that emerges from the cocoon.

CHAPTER THIRTY-THREE

The Plan to Escape

The cocoon started to rattle. CUE "EYE OF THE TIGER" MUSIC. I was planning to break out of my cocoon. My idea: Get back on my feet at SeaWorld. Preparation: Hire a swim coach to make sure I could pass the swim test. Goal: Full-time job, steady pay, benefits, and breaking free from the cocoon.

It had been a while since I had been swimming, and I wanted to make sure I was in the best shape for the swim test. I practiced daily with a swim coach and felt stronger and more physically fit than I had in a long time. I applied to SeaWorld and received an invitation to take the swim test in a month. The plan was coming together. What could possibly go wrong?

One day I was feeling a little sick and decided to get a massage. The masseuse warned me that when people are feeling sick, a massage could either make them feel better or worse. Nonsense! I would feel better.

Hello, bronchitis! Apparently the masseuse was right. It could make me feel worse. I went from not feeling great to full blown bronchitis in no time. I went to the emergency room twice, was given cortisone shots and antibiotics each time to help me get better, but nothing helped. I was coughing uncontrollably and felt tightness in my chest. It was getting worse. Before I knew it, the time had arrived to fly out to California to take the test, and I was still very sick.

I arranged to fly into Los Angeles, rent a car, then... get ready for this... take a two hour drive up to Ventura where my doctor was, get medication to take care of the bronchitis - I didn't have health insurance in Hawaii, so I needed to go to my doctor in Ventura - then drive all the way down to San Diego, about a four hour drive. The swim test was in less than twenty-four hours. I was exhausted and really sick. I talked to Christine, my friend who got the full-time SeaWorld job at the same time as I did.

"Joy, you can't do it. You'll get pneumonia. That water is in the 60's. It's not worth it," she said. I thought about not doing it, but I couldn't use this as an excuse. I had to go for it, bronchitis and all. BRING UP "EYE OF THE TIGER" MUSIC.

The next day I was at SeaWorld with a group of healthy applicants ready to take the test. "Is anyone here sick?" my old boss asked the group. I hesitantly raised my hand.

"But you're not *that* sick, right?"

"Right," I sheepishly responded. He knew that I couldn't take the test if I were sick, and then my opportunity to come back would be gone. I have to say I was hoping for an out. "Oh, you're sick? Here is a waiver for this part of the audition process," but that just didn't happen.

The underwater breath hold was difficult for a healthy person, much less someone who was coughing uncontrollably every other minute. I just had to visualize. Just relax and visualize. They picked me to go in the first group. *I can do this,* I thought. I looked across the pool to the end. I visualized how far I needed to go and that I would want to quit and take a breath of air, but I wouldn't. *Let's do this.* I dove in and started singing, *Borderline, seems like I'm going to lose my mind. You just keep on pushing my love, over the borderline.*

I felt myself pull and kick fast. I needed to get through the water. I felt the need for oxygen and didn't think I could make it. Suddenly I was passing center stage. I was half way there. I needed air.

You keep on pushing my love... over the borderline.

Okay, there is the light from the gate, I'm ALMOST there. Just a few more strokes and I can start ascending. I started my slow ascent, and before I knew it, I was at the end. I made it! Holy smokes! It took everything out of me. I had used up every ounce of energy to take the test so I stayed in the water for a minute. My legs were like Jello. They felt like they would collapse if I tried to get out of the pool at that moment. I had been bed ridden for a month before the test trying to get well. My body went from 0 to 60 and was trying to catch up. After a brief rest I got out of the pool and walked back to the other side. Next I had to dive off of the bridge. My feet felt like frozen rocks that were detached from my body. I climbed up on top of the rock bridge, which was no easy task because I couldn't feel my feet. The supervisor was there to help people. She said, "Not bad for a girl with bronchitis," and smiled at me. *Yeah! I did it! I can't feel my feet and may be in the process of developing pneumonia, but I did it!*

I passed the swim test so I thought the rest was in the bag. They knew me. They loved me. I got the job! I called my family to let them know the good news. I hadn't had my interview yet, but I was sure that my only obstacle was the swim test, and I passed that. The rest was easy sailing.

When I walked into the interview, I sat there with some people I had known and worked with before and a person from HR. My friends were very professional and did a great job of acting impartial. Then the HR questions came up. You know, "Tell me a time when you had a problem with a co-worker and how you were able to resolve it," the typical HR questions. I nailed this part before, but this time my examples were from working in a restaurant, and I was too embarrassed to use those answers so I tried to remember examples from five years prior when I was working at SeaWorld. Did I mention that I had a lot of chemo and my memory wasn't the greatest? I couldn't think of examples from five years ago. It was just fuzzy. In addition, I was sick and on medication, so I committed the cardinal sin of responding with "Pass." As if that weren't bad enough, I responded with "Pass" more than once!

I left SeaWorld thinking that the interview wasn't great, but I still thought that I had the job. I started my journey back to Hawaii. I had a two-hour drive ahead of me to get to the Los Angeles airport. That's when I got a call from my former boss.

"Unfortunately, we aren't able to offer you a full-time job, but I am able to offer you a seasonal position," he said.

"Okay. Really? It was my interview wasn't it?" I asked.

"It was the interview and after the underwater swim, it took you awhile to get out of the water."

My heart sank. All of that work, preparation, risk of pneumonia, and I didn't get the job! I had never been a seasonal employee. I was always employed with a full-time job. This meant that I would be employed for the summer, and that was it. I could possibly be moving from Hawaii to San Diego only to work for the summer and then... unemployment. I was devastated. Just devastated. Still it was a chance to get back on my feet. Hopefully they would hire me when a full-time position became available later on. He gave me time to think about it before giving my answer.

In all honesty it was kind of embarrassing to come back as a "seasonal," but I really wanted/needed this in my life. My friends from SeaWorld were devastated for me and said, "You aren't going to take it are you?" Well, the only one it would hurt if I refused the position would be me, so I swallowed my pride and said "Yes," hoping that I could get a full-time job in the future.

That evening I made a phone call to Bailey. Her mom answered and told me that she had some friends over, but that she would love to talk to me. I waited as she got Bailey. I could hear kids playing in the background. It had been four years since we were in the hospital together, fighting for our lives. Now we were both on the other side of cancer. I loved that she was a normal kid again. I loved knowing that she was with her friends. Then I heard the phone pick up and Bailey said, "Hi!"

It's hard to explain, but it sounded like more than a greeting. It was more like she was on the phone with someone who knew what she had gone through, who had been through it too. She was with her friends now, and things were good, but we had been through an experience together that most cannot imagine. It was that kind of, "Hi," the kind that spoke volumes.

"Hi, Bailey! How are you?" I asked.

"Good," she said. I could feel her smile from over the phone.

"I just got a job working with the dolphins again at SeaWorld."

"You did?" she said.

"Yes, and you know what that means? You can come down here, and I will introduce you to a dolphin. Would you like that?"

"Yes!"

She was excited! It felt so good to talk to her. We battled cancer at the same time, and we had both made it. Now, years later, I could finally have her come to SeaWorld to meet a dolphin. I was on the road back to a stable life. One foot broke free of the cocoon.

CHAPTER THIRTY-FOUR

SeaWorld, Take Two

Being back at SeaWorld felt good. I was getting steady paychecks, and I wasn't killing myself for every dime that I made. On one of my first days back I got to sit down on the rocks and watch someone swim with a dolphin. I couldn't believe how lucky I was. I wasn't running around a restaurant because it was frowned upon to stop moving. I wasn't schlepping drinks or talking to a salty bartender. I wasn't serving tourists who seemed nice but gave horrible tips and stayed way too long. Things were different now. I could take a breath and look around, kiss a dolphin, go for a swim, and the whole time I was getting paid!

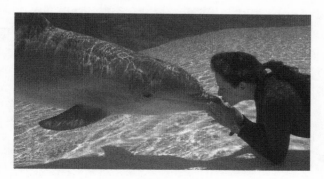

My home life was still a mixed bag consisting of good, not so good, and what am I doing? Dave and I were living together. He had moved to San Diego to attend law school. At one point he started talking about signing another lease together, and for some reason I decided to put my foot down.

"I'm not going to sign another lease unless we are engaged or married." Why did I say this? Because I wanted things to either go somewhere or end (I don't know if I really thought it would end). All I knew was that for four and a half years we had been together. I had stuck it out, sold everything I owned, moved to Hawaii, and lived in poverty. We were still together, and he hadn't asked me to marry him. Don't you think that after four and a half years he would be able to make a decision on a relationship? This was certainly no fairytale that I had ever seen or imagined. I felt like I had put a lot of years in, and I "deserved" a marriage proposal.

Let's get back to my ballsy moment of, "I'm not going to sign another lease unless we are engaged or married."

He was shocked at my statement.

"Well, you have to give me some time to think about it," he said.

Maybe he needs time so that he can ask me to marry him in the right way, I thought.

Then one night he told me what his decision was. He hemmed and hawed. Then finally the truth came out.

"It's just that I've never pictured myself getting married," he said.

My heart sank. This was not the proposal I was expecting.

"I just never pictured myself getting married - to anyone – ever," he said.

Oh, I feel better, I thought. *You don't want to marry anybody, ever. You didn't feel compelled to tell me that at any point during those four and half years we were together?*

Then he said the craziest thing to explain his decision.

"It's just that I've always pictured myself dying alone."

"I hope you get your wish," I said, a little proud of my quick retort to his absurd statement.

Now you may be asking yourself "Did he ever allude to marriage or were you just delusional?" Well, he did in fact allude to marriage. He had said years before that he would not get me a diamond ring because of blood diamonds so it would probably be a sapphire. I considered this a clue that he would propose to me with a sapphire. He also talked to me about marriage when I moved to Hawaii. I freaked out a few days after arriving because I was risking my health insurance by being there. He told me we could get married so that I would be covered by his health insurance. I told him I didn't want to get married because of health insurance. I wanted to marry for love. I assumed that he would eventually ask me, but the whole, "I always pictured myself dying alone" thing never came up.

Back at SeaWorld things were good. I was offered a full-time position in the animal training department. The only full-time position after the summer was at a place called Rocky Point. It was an area I wasn't familiar with, and I felt like I didn't know what I was doing. At this point some of the euphoria started to wear off.

While working at Rocky Point I met so many great people. All of the people who worked there were very close and would always do things together outside of work. It was exactly what I needed since I was trying to get over Dave. I could hang out with my new group of friends and not sit at home feeling sorry for myself. The healthiest thing was for me to be around other people, and it worked. I started to feel whole again. I started to feel like me. It was the first time since I finished the chemotherapy that I felt like the person I was before, strong Joy.

Time flew by, and before I knew it, another group was applying for the seasonal summer positions. One of the seasonals who came to our area was a guy named Alex who had worked in another department at SeaWorld. Before I ever met him, I heard about him. Apparently he wanted to work at Rocky Point so that he could "hook up" with all the girls. At least that is what some girl said in the locker room as she was gossiping (and you know how reliable that information is).

Months passed by, and I didn't pay attention to him at all. Then one day we had to work together. There were two dolphins, a male and a female, that were stuck to one another. They were stuck to each other because the female was cycling, and the male, well the male was just being a male, which meant he wouldn't leave her side. A cycling female is hard for a male to resist. The female, Cometta, would turn on her side with her eyes closed, and the male, Crunch, would just sit there underneath her. Alex and I were up for a training session together. The goal: to feed Cometta and Crunch when they left each other, if only for a brief period of time. At least it would be a start.

I loved the challenge! I had the female, Cometta, and Alex had the male, Crunch. I told him my plan to be able to walk away with Cometta for a little bit and feed her when she left, then come back to Crunch before he left Alex. We started our session. Everything was great. Cometta and I would leave for a bit. Then I would yell out to Alex to cross my path with Crunch, and before I knew it, he was doing things before I asked. We were getting success. It was wonderful. It was as if he could read what my next move was, and then he knew exactly what to do. The session ended. Success! We were able to reinforce them for leaving each other! And, oddly enough, we were a great team. Afterward I walked up to him and said, "That was great!" I was excited and a bit out of breath from running around. "I loved how you anticipated what had to be done. I didn't even have to ask you. That was a great session!"

Now I don't know why, but I stopped talking after that. I turned and walked away. It may have been because we were both out of breath, smiling from ear to ear, and looking at each other. He had a huge smile on his face, and for some reason I just stopped talking and left. Sometimes I cannot explain my socially awkward moments.

By this time Dave and I had been broken up for eight months. Every once in a while we would hang out. He would tell me that he missed me and wanted to get back together. He brought me flowers, wine, chocolates, pretty much anything he thought I would like. He would talk about how there wasn't anyone else like me (the cancer survivor, dolphin trainer, filmmaker thing was a difficult combination to find, or at least that is what he would tell me. I think he was probably right). I wasn't interested. I was finally doing the right thing.

Then one night he called and really wanted to see me. I tried to get out of it but ended up agreeing to see him. I met him outside of my apartment. He brought me roses (first time in four and a half years, while complaining about how much they cost), specialty beer (how romantic), and a hand written note telling me that he would be honored to "wear a ring to signify our love." After all of this time, after all of the heartache and heartbreak, he told me he wanted to marry me. This was the reason why we had broken up eight months ago. It was what I thought I wanted when I was with him, to take the next step, but now I realized that this would have been a huge mistake, and I would have been settling.

"No, a thousand times no. If you had come to me eight months ago, I would have said yes but now it is a thousand times no," I said.

The cycle of breaking up and getting back together was finally broken, and I passed the final test. He knew he did everything he could to get me back. He even asked me to "wear a ring to signify our love," and I didn't budge. It was over. I felt so strong for being able to say this. I felt like the old Joy. I had emerged from the cocoon, whole and strong.

CHAPTER THIRTY-FIVE

Magic

I believe in magic. Does that sound silly? I believe in those magical moments in life that seem like they belong in a movie, those moments that seem too good to be true. Once I had gone to a David Copperfield show, and I was picked out of the audience to be a part of his magic trick. He was going to make a group of people disappear. Ahhh, how exciting until... the lights dimmed, a sheet covered us, and a voice from the darkness said, "Everyone stand up and exit to your left." We were led off of the stage and into a holding area in the back. LAME! I didn't disappear and reappear on a tropical island. I walked off the stage. Don't ever show me a magic trick again. I want to be wowed, and I really want to believe in magic.

More than a silly magic trick that wows a crowd, I love everyday magical moments. The night that Dave proposed I had a magical moment. I suppose it was magical that I had the strength to say no. It was because I said no that life gave me the most wonderful magical gift.

After I said no to Dave, I had two choices: stay home or go out with my friends. Normally I would choose to stay home, but on this day I chose to go out with my friends. Being alone and letting myself ruminate about

Dave would not have been a good idea. I jumped in a taxi and went downtown to meet up with a group of friends from Rocky Point.

When I arrived at the club, things started out great. The bouncer complimented me on my perfume (it was just lotion). Then as I walked in, the song "I Can't Wait" by Nu Shoos was playing. I loved that song, probably because it brought me back to when I was younger and would make mixed tapes from the songs that played on the radio. I would get just as excited if they played, "Don't Want To Fall In Love" by Jane Child.

"I love this song!" I said as I walked up.

Alex was standing with the group and said, "I was just saying that!"

What a line, I thought. There is no way he could actually like this song.

"Whatever!" I eloquently replied to him.

"No, really! I was just saying that."

I looked at him suspiciously but then thought maybe he really does like this song. I mean it made me really happy. I couldn't be the only one.

I danced with my girlfriends for a while and then took a break. That's when I started talking to Alex.

"Would you like to dance?" he asked.

"Sure," I said.

We all danced together and had a great time at Rocky Point parties. We went onto the dance floor. He held me close. I always liked dancing close because there is less chance of me looking like an idiot when I dance. One song after another came on, and we were still dancing together. At one point I realized that we were dancing with our foreheads touching, and we were looking into each other's eyes. *Oh my gosh, how long have we been doing that?* I wondered. I felt like I should have been uncomfortable, but I wasn't. I didn't want to pull away once I realized we were gazing into each other's eyes. It felt like we had been doing it for an eternity, and I could continue doing it for an eternity. It was magic, real life magic (the best kind).

As the night went on, some friends noticed the weird scene that was unfolding. My girlfriend, L.J., came up to me and whispered in a drunk, trying to be discreet, but incredibly loud voice, "Do *you* need help?"

"No, I'm good. Thanks," I replied.

Alex dipped me. I LOVE being dipped! After a while I noticed that whenever he dipped me, I'd hear a sound. One time when he dipped me, I looked to see what the sound was. He was kissing my jawbone whenever he'd dip me, but it was so light that I hadn't noticed... or maybe it was the tequila. *Wow, that is pretty gutsy to kiss me,* I thought. Before I knew it, the night was over, the club was closing, and we were all leaving. Alex offered to drive me home.

"I'm surprised you're single," he said.

"I know, but I was proposed to tonight! I just said no," I said in an attempt to let him know that there was nothing wrong with me. I just hadn't found the right one.

Now I have a history of when I'm on a date with someone (not that this was an official date), I do this really weird thing at the end of the night. I make every effort possible to avoid the "end of the night kiss." "Why?" you might ask. Because it is so predictable and boring! I want to be swept off my feet. Kiss me in the middle of the date, not at the end. I had this "Joy Move" that I would do as my date dropped me off.

As we approached my house, I would unbuckle my seatbelt so I was ready to exit, and the minute the car stopped (and sometimes as it was still rolling) I would open the car door and jump out, thanking my date for a great night while he looked at me like, "What just happened?" Thus, successful avoidance of the much-anticipated "end of the night kiss." I would giggle to myself as I walked away. If someone really liked me, he would have to be smart enough to figure this out.

Alex came to a stop, and I still had my seatbelt on. This was huge! I really liked him. My escape instinct didn't kick in. I unbuckled my seatbelt and waited for what seemed like an eternity compared to any other date. In real time it was about five seconds. Then the instinct kicked in, and before I knew it, I was out of the car saying goodbye. I had accidentally activated the "Joy Move" because I was in a stopped car in front of my house. I wish I had stayed a little longer. It was the best night of my life.

Whenever I met someone that I was interested in, I wondered how he would react to finding out that I survived cancer. The guy I was dating while I found out that I was sick did not do well with the news. I didn't want that to happen again so I needed to see what Alex's reaction would be when he found out I had been sick.

A few days after our magical night, Alex and I worked together. We walked by the water on rocks that were slick with algae. He took a big step to get to another rock, then turned around and reached out his hand to help me across. He was being a gentleman, but instead of taking his hand, I jumped across the rocks on my own. Then I looked at him and said, "You know, I'm stronger than you think," he smiled at me.

"Did you know that I survived cancer?"

"No, I didn't know that. Are you okay now?" he looked concerned.

"I'm great. I even made a documentary on my battle with cancer. There is a trailer for it on my MySpace page if you want to see it." (Yes, I know no one uses that anymore, but at the time it was THE thing to do).

"I would love to see it. I'll watch it tonight," he said.

Okay, okay he seemed fine when I mentioned it. He didn't seem freaked out by it, but only time would tell. I waited for him to pull away from me, especially after seeing me sick and bald in the video.

The next day when I saw Alex, he said, "I watched your film, and I love your story!" Not only was he not freaked out, but he seemed even more interested in me. Okay, he passed the test!

Our time working together was about to end. He was offered a full-time job working as a marine mammal trainer for the Navy. His last week at SeaWorld flew by, and before I knew it, he was gone. He hadn't asked me out. I guess it was just one night of magic, and that was all it would ever be. I mean he was seven and a half years younger than I was. It wouldn't have worked out anyway. There would be nothing to talk about, nothing in common, but the only thing was that I had never felt like that before in my life. I had never felt such a connection with someone just dancing.

He came back to work one day to return a key, but by the time I could talk to him he was gone. Then I got a message from him on MySpace.

"It was good seeing you today," he said.

That was it.

I wrote back, "You should have stayed. I didn't have a chance to talk to you."

He wrote back, "I would like to take you to lunch if you are free this weekend."

But by this time I had all of these doubts that crept into my mind. What did we have in common? And that age difference was insane. What was I thinking?

The next day I talked to one of my co-workers about it. I told him I wasn't sure whether or not I should go out with Alex.

"Well, I probably shouldn't be telling you this, but a few months ago Alex and I were talking about who we would date at SeaWorld," he said as I cringed. I didn't want to hear about the girls Alex would date... yuck.

"Alex said, 'If there is one person I could fall in love with at SeaWorld, it's Joy.'"

"Wait, when was that?" I asked.

"Oh, this was a few months ago."

Alex had said that months before our magical night. Okay, I'll go on the date. "Thank you, God, for these everyday magical moments. They make life so much better!"

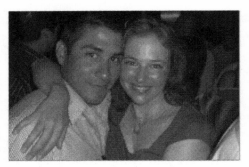

CHAPTER THIRTY-SIX

The Date

I t's lunch, just lunch so if it goes horribly wrong, then it was just lunch. What if we have nothing in common and nothing to talk about, and then the magic is gone. He took me out to lunch in Old Town, a part of San Diego that is known for its Mexican food. At the worst I would have a wonderful meal in Old Town.

How in the world would our conversation go for our first official date? This could be a really uncomfortable lunch while we find out that we have absolutely nothing in common. Then Alex started to talk. He had a ton of incredible stories about his childhood, being in the military, being an army ranger, going to Afghanistan, and living in Hawaii. That is right. He lived in Hawaii! That was where he was stationed in the military, AND we were in Hawaii at the same time for a couple of months! I could have walked by him in Waikiki or stood next to him one night while watching the fireworks. Lunch went so well! In fact, I didn't want the date to end. I guess he didn't either.

"Do you want to go for a walk?" he asked.

"Yes!" I said, excited that I could spend some more time with him.

He drove up the coast to Del Mar, and we went for a walk on the beach and just talked the whole time. We talked about everything.

"Do you want to have kids?" he asked. The truth was that I didn't know if I could have kids, so I avoided the question.

I felt like I was being interviewed for a position as his wife. This was crazy. I asked Alex about what I had heard regarding him wanting to work at Rocky Point so that he could date all of the girls there. That was the one thing that made me wonder about him. He shook his head.

"I said that to my co-workers because I was trying to make light of the fact that I was leaving them to go to another department," he said.

That actually made sense. Okay, that works for me.

We walked until we ran out of beach. He saved me from a stray football that almost hit me, though I never saw it. I just saw him scramble in front of me and catch something. I thought he was showboating, but apparently he saved me!

When we reached his jeep, he looked at me and said, "You know, I always thought I would fall for a girl with curly brown hair and green eyes."

That's me! Wait a minute... was that a line? I don't care! I think I love him! It was the most wonderful first date of my life.

CHAPTER THIRTY-SEVEN

Bailey

There are moments in life that touch us, and moments that we will never forget. The moment that I met my five-year-old roommate, Bailey, at Children's Hospital Los Angeles was a moment that I will never forget. She had a shining smile and was beyond adorable. She also had leukemia. Kids get cancer too. When I was at Children's Hospital, I got to see all of the brave kids who battled cancer. They showed me what it really meant to be strong.

I set up a time and date for Bailey to come down to SeaWorld to meet a dolphin. I paid for it with my credit card. It cost me a lot of money, but it was worth it. Then maybe a day or two before she was supposed to come to SeaWorld, I found out that it wasn't going to happen. There had been a miscommunication. Her mom thought I was going to babysit Bailey and her older sister while at SeaWorld. I couldn't, I was working that day. My dream of the two of us getting in the water and meeting a dolphin after surviving cancer would have to wait.

Time went by, and before I knew it, a year had passed. One of the things that I wrote on my "to do" list was to bring Bailey back for a dolphin interaction. I really wanted her to meet a dolphin. It didn't work out the first time, but we would make it happen this time, and there wouldn't be any confusion. The last time I spoke to Bailey and her mom, she was a normal kid, growing up, going to school, going to birthday parties, and doing other normal "kid things." She had been through the wringer, and now she was getting her childhood back.

One evening I was walking to my car when I got a phone call. I didn't recognize the phone number. I wasn't going to pick it up. Then at the last moment I decided to see who it was.

"Joy?" a woman on the line asked.

"Yes? Who is this?"

"It's Bailey's mom."

"Hi!" I was instantly happy to hear her voice. She had been on my mind to call so I could get them back down to San Diego.

"I can't believe it. I can't believe I found your phone number. I was just cleaning her room, and I found your phone number."

Okay, that explained why I hadn't heard from them in a while.

"I have some bad news... Bailey is gone," she said.

"What do you mean?" I was hoping that she had the worst way of expressing herself, and Bailey was at a sleepover or camp or something.

"Bailey passed away a couple of days ago."

This couldn't be happening. This wasn't how it was supposed to work out.

"I thought that she was doing well? She was in remission. Wasn't she in remission?" I asked.

Her mom told me that Bailey's cancer came back. I remember certain words or phrases like "another bone marrow transplant," and "her little body just couldn't take it anymore, she had enough." She passed away in her mom's arms, in the hospital.

Why her? Why not me? She shouldn't have had to go through this! I waited too long to invite her back! I didn't know! It was on my list! Why didn't I call her earlier? I didn't know she was sick again. I would have gone to see her in a second, I thought frantically, unable to believe that this had happened.

"Bailey asked for you," she said.

"She did?" My heart dropped.

"Yeah, she did. I couldn't find your phone number so I called SeaWorld and left a message for you. I told her it was really important. I even remember the name of the person I spoke to," she said. Apparently she got a different department. The message never got to me. My heart broke into a million pieces, a million devastated pieces. *Bailey asked for me? I can't believe she asked for me, and I wasn't there!* I thought as I cried uncontrollably.

Her mom invited me to Bailey's memorial. The one request was that I wear a sundress. She wanted it to be a celebration of her life. She knew Bailey wouldn't want people to be sad for her so she threw a big party. It was about a four-hour drive for me to get to her memorial. It was off of a dirt road, and there were colorful balloons and kids playing by a pond, a bar-b-q, and lots of sundresses. There were easily over a hundred people there. It was a beautiful sunny hot day. I stood there and watched kids her age run around the grass in their bare feet playing games. Some were swimming. Some were walking around with plates full of food. They were all having fun. I imagined Bailey there playing in the pond or running around with bare feet in the grass, but I knew that she was in a better place, a place where she would never be sick again. It was a wonderful celebration of life and a moment that will be with me for the rest of my life.

CHAPTER THIRTY-EIGHT

The Dream Reimagined

Some people come into our lives for a reason, whether it is to open our eyes to another world, or to make us appreciate what we have, or even to break our hearts so that we will forever be impacted by them. I believe Alex came into my life to help heal me with love and to motivate me with his own unstoppable spirit. He not only made me happier than I had been in my entire life, but he motivated me. He was always setting goals that others thought were unachievable, almost laughable, until he actually achieved them. He believed in himself, and he believed in me.

One day we drove down to Ensenada to have lunch. We found a little restaurant where we sat down to have fish tacos. We started talking about our dreams.

"I want to fight in the UFC (Ultimate Fighting Championship) on a pay-per-view card. What about you? Do you have a dream?" he asked.

"Hmm…" I said. I had a dream. It was my dream to have Bailey come down to SeaWorld to meet a dolphin, but that would never happen now. I tried to quickly come up with a replacement dream, but I couldn't. All I could think about was Bailey. "Well… I've had this dream that I just can't stop thinking about. I wanted to have Bailey, my roommate from Children's Hospital, come to SeaWorld. I wanted her to be able to get into the water with me and then I could introduce her to a dolphin. I've had this dream since I was in the hospital, but I can't make it happen. She died. I just can't stop thinking about it," I said as I held back tears and gave a helpless shrug with my shoulders.

"Well, maybe you don't have to give up that dream."

"Of course I do. She died before I could make it happen."

"I know you can't have her meet a dolphin, but it doesn't mean your dream has to die," he said. I took a drink and tried to compose myself. It was hard talking about Bailey. "Maybe you can do something more, like have an event where you bring kids with cancer to SeaWorld, and they can meet a dolphin. I know it's not Bailey, but it would make a big difference in the lives of so many other kids. She'll always be your inspiration."

"That's a great idea. I love it!"

"See, you don't need to give up on your dreams," he said with a smile.

"Okay, when I get home I'll write up a proposal and see what they say."

Now, I just needed to approach SeaWorld about it. I didn't know how they would react. I mean I was proposing to give away free interactions. How in the world could that go over well? My idea was to do the interactions during the off-season when there were fewer people in the park. I basically thought of any reason why they might say no and came up with a justification for them to say yes. I wrote up a one-page proposal and approached my boss with it. When he finished reading it, he looked up at me. I was ready to blurt out all of the reasons why this could work. Then my boss started to talk.

"I love it!" he said. I was caught off guard, I had prepared to rebut with a solution to any problem that he came up with.

"Really?" I replied.

"Yeah, this is a great idea. It's a no-brainer."

He immediately made some phone calls while I was still there and got the ball rolling. I asked Dr. Siegel to write the requirements necessary for a patient to participate in the program. Dr. Siegel did that and also gave me the name of a doctor to contact at Rady Children's Hospital in San Diego. This doctor could get me in contact with the right people to start the program with their hospital. My cold call to them felt very strange.

"Yeah, um, I am a patient of Dr. Siegel's from Children's Hospital Los Angeles, and I want to provide dolphin interactions for patients going through cancer..."

It sounded weird, but I got through to the right people and our first annual Rady Children's Hospital event was scheduled a few months after Bailey's memorial. I was so happy that we had this event for Rady's, but I also wanted kids from the hospital where I was treated, Children's Hospital Los Angeles, to be able to meet a dolphin too. SeaWorld once again said "Yes." They also provided two additional tickets to enter the park for family members so that they could watch their child enjoy the interaction and also gave the hospital a CD of the photos to give out to the families. It was wonderful. I was so grateful.

A big part of these interactions was not only meeting a dolphin but knowing a little bit of my story. That may sound silly, but I wanted to show them that I was happy, healthy, and living my dream. I think that was a very important part of the interactions. It was about more than meeting a dolphin, which was beyond cool. It was about giving hope. It was showing an example of someone who had battled cancer, followed her dream, and who was giving back. Wouldn't it be wonderful if they grew up and gave back too? It would be a wonderful full circle story.

The first year I was too afraid to say anything. I had read somewhere not to talk about your experiences so I went against my gut. I thought they knew that I was a cancer survivor too, but I soon started to realize that they had no idea who I was. They thought I was just a trainer.

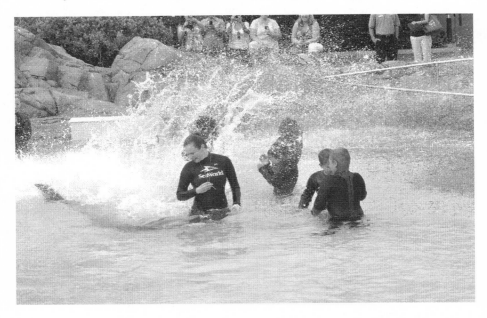

During one event I was waiting to get in the water with some of the kids who were battling cancer from Children's Hospital Los Angeles. There was a boy in the group who was about five years old. He had no hair, a big smile, and an even bigger personality. He had his arms folded as we waited to get in the water. I watched as he took in everything that was happening, the dolphins, the wetsuit, the sand. He would ask questions with confidence. Then he turned to me and said in a matter-of-fact way, "Do you know that I have leukemia?" I looked at him and then got down low so I could be at his level.

"Do you know that I had cancer too?" I asked. He shook his head as he focused on me. "Yeah, I had cancer about 10 years ago. It was a blood cancer, just like you, and I was treated at a Children's Hospital Los Angeles just like you. Now, look…" I said as I looked at the dolphins. "I get to work here at my dream job, and I get to share it with you," I said as I pointed at him. His eyes lit up. As I began to stand up, I could see his parents in the background smiling and wiping away tears.

From that moment on during every Children's Hospital event, I would make sure to let the kids know a little bit about my story. Right before we got into the water, I turned to the group of kids, clad in wet-suits and said, "My name is Joy, and I know a lot of you have been treated at Children's Hospital. I was too. About eleven years ago I had cancer, and now I am working at my dream job here at SeaWorld. I wanted to share what I get to do every day with you."

It was the best way I had of saying it without saying too much. Then a little boy said, "I have cancer too! Mine is bone cancer. What kind did you have?" he asked.

"I had non-Hodgkin's lymphoma," I told him.

Then another kid said, "I have leukemia. I just try to be positive every day."

I heard other kids say what they had. I didn't ask them to tell me. They just wanted to. It was an everyday magical moment.

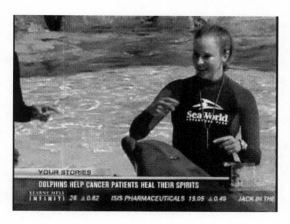

CHAPTER THIRTY-NINE

My Fairytale

One day Alex said, "I am so thankful for Dave."

I looked at him as though he had lost his mind.

"Why would you say that?" I asked.

"Because Dave kept you off the market until I could find you. If it weren't for him, you would probably be married by now," he said.

It was the best possible way to look at the reason why Dave had been a part of my journey. Four and a half years that I thought had led to nothing had really led me to my soulmate.

Alex was the most wonderful boyfriend. He made me so happy and always told me how happy I made him and how lucky he felt. One day Alex came over to see me after work.

"You know, I had butterflies when I knew I was going to see you today," he said with a big smile.

"Really? Butterflies?"

"Yeah, I had that feeling in my stomach on my way over here."

"Oh stop it! We've been dating for a year! Did you really feel like that?"

"I really did," he said. Magic.

My parents told me it was the happiest and the most at peace that they had ever seen me.

Alex encouraged me to finish my documentary that I had been sitting on for so long. I finally finished in 2008 and submitted "Just One Year –A story of triumph over cancer" to film festivals.

"Dad, I got an email from the film festival," I said over the phone.

"Yes…" he said.

"I didn't get in," I said to him, trying to contain my excitement.

"Oh, I'm sorry, Honey."

"Just kidding! I got in!"

"What? Really?" he asked.

"Really! I got accepted, and they will be showing my documentary as part of their festival!"

"You can't scare me like that!" he said while laughing. "Joy, I'm so proud of you. That is just incredible!"

Before I knew it, my documentary was accepted to four film festivals.

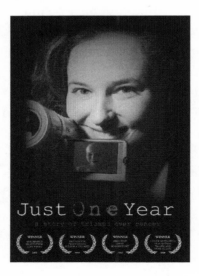

Then one day at work I got a call from my stepmom.

"Joy, where are you?" she asked.

"I'm at work. Why?"

"I need you to sit down."

"Why? What happened?" I asked as I lowered myself to the ground to sit.

"Your dad had a stroke. It's pretty bad, Joy."

I was at work, sitting on the ground in my wetsuit sobbing.

I jumped on a plane to be by his side. I can only say it was one of the hardest things that I have ever gone through. We had to take him off of life support. My dad knew that I was happy with Alex, but he never had a chance to meet him or even talk to him. Alex called to check on me as I sat by my dad's side at the hospital.

"Would it be okay if I talked to him?" he asked.

"Um, yeah, you want to do that?"

"Yes."

"Okay, here I'm putting the phone to his ear."

My dad was off of life support at this time so the room was silent. Then Alex started to talk and I could hear everything.

"Hello, sir. I really wish I had the chance to meet you. I'm sorry this happened. I just wanted you to know that I really love your daughter, and I'm going to take good care of her for the rest of her life, so you don't have to worry," he said. Tears were falling from my face as I tried to be quiet. "It was nice meeting you, sir. I hope you have a safe journey."

I brought the phone back to my ear. "I love you so much, Alex."

Sometimes we have to go through broken roads, wrong turns, and speed bumps to find the right path and the right person. Alex was the right person.

"Thank you, God, for Alex."

On Valentine's Day we drove to Julian with his dog, Charly, to see the snow and go on a hike. Alex found a large tree that had fallen over and climbed onto the snowy log, then reached out his hand to help me climb up there with him. After I climbed up, Alex pointed to Charly who was behind me. "Look at him. He is loving the snow," he said. I turned to look and saw Charly, a red colored English cocker spaniel, happily hopping through the snow. When I turned back, Alex was down on one knee on the snowy log with an open ring box and inside was a beautiful diamond ring.

"Will you marry me?" he asked.

"Yes!" I said.

I am so lucky that I found him and so lucky that Dave kept me occupied until Alex could find me.

When I told Ann about Alex's proposal the first thing she said was, "Congratulations!" which was quickly followed by, "This means I get to help you pick out a wedding dress! I love trying on wedding dresses!"

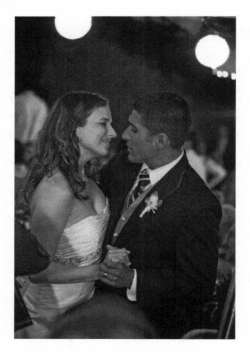

Alex and I got married in Del Mar above the same beach where we went for a long walk on our first date and he asked me if I wanted to have kids. Our reception was absolutely beautiful. It was in his parents' backyard, and his dad custom built strands of lights that he strung over the backyard and we hung colored lanterns on each light. L.J. (the girl who asked if I needed help when Alex and I danced together for the first time), helped me decorate the backyard with more lights, candles, luminaries, and flowers. At our wedding we were surrounded by friends and family. Some of the same people who had been with me when I was sick were there at our wedding. My mom, Aunt Susan, Uncle David, Kevin, and Ann were just some of the many people who were there on my wedding day and who had also been with me throughout my battle with cancer.

At the reception Kevin got up to give a speech.

"Hello, everybody, my name is Kevin, and I've been a friend of Joy's for about eight years now. We went to film school together. In that time period eight years ago several people and I in this room undertook a mission to save a girl's life." My stomach tightened, and I felt a flood of emotion rush over me. I turned my head and locked eyes with Ann. She ran up and brought me a tissue. Kevin continued:

"And, I think it's because we were all greedy, and we didn't want to see or have this beautiful girl taken away from us. At that point in time there was somebody in her life that wasn't worthy of her love, her smile, and her warmth, but to me that goes to show that there are no coincidences, and that things happen for a reason. Those six months were some of the toughest times for all of us, but it was all worth it to see her standing here today, smiling brighter than I've ever seen her smile. I think I can speak for all of us, that we're in the fight with you, Joy, that we still have your back. Now I extend that to Alex and welcome him as a friend because it's nice to see that she has finally found someone who is worthy of her love, smile, and warmth."

Kevin's speech really hit home. It put this wonderful moment in the context of what we had all been through, everything that my friends and family had fought for and how truly special it was that we were all celebrating eight years later at my wedding.

"Thank you, God, for the wonderful people in my life. I truly feel blessed."

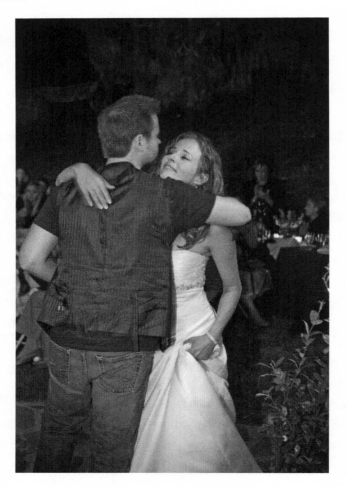

CHAPTER FORTY

Two Passes

"Who are you here to see?" asked the person at the front desk. "Dr. Siegel," I said.

The receptionist wrote something on two passes and handed them both to me. I looked at the two passes before I took them from her. I'd never received two.

I'd been coming to Children's Hospital Los Angeles for over a decade to see Dr. Siegel. First it was for chemotherapy. Then it was for annual checkups that I will have for the rest of my life. It's amazing how much things can change - how your position in life, your outlook, and your life can change. It was over a decade ago that I was getting my one sticker to go to Four East where I would stay for five days and receive chemotherapy in hopes that it would save my life. It was over a decade ago that my friends were helping me walk through these same halls because I was so weak from the chemotherapy that my legs were buckling when I tried to walk. This time I was at Children's Hospital for my annual checkup. I grabbed the two passes and put one on my jacket. The second one went on my nine-month-old daughter's sweater.

Christiana Joy Soto is the most incredible little girl I could have ever imagined or asked for. We were told that it was highly unlikely that I would be able to have a child. My follicle-stimulating hormone (FSH) was very high, which meant that my chances were very low. I was close to menopause. We met with a specialist to see if she had any advice. She took blood samples and performed an ultrasound on the first appointment. She told us it didn't look good, but we had to wait for the blood work to come back to know if she could help us have a child.

By the time the second appointment came, Alex and I found out that I was pregnant. We went into the appointment excited to tell our doctor. She looked quite serious as she started telling us the results of the test. It wasn't good news. I wasn't even a good candidate for in vitro. Alex and I looked at each other knowing that what she said didn't matter at this point. "I'm pregnant!" I happily exclaimed.

I held my daughter in my arms as I walked to the oncology clinic. She started to pull the sticker off and attempted to eat it. She had no idea what her mommy had been through to get to this point. The emotions welled up inside of me as I carried her through the same hallways I had walked through so many times before as I fought for my life and watched others fight for their lives. It didn't escape me how fortunate we were. We were healthy. I held my little girl closer and gave her kisses on her cheek. I knew what a blessing good health was. I thought of Bailey and all that she had gone through at such a young age. All I could think about was how grateful I was for my health and for my daughter's health. My checkup went well. I was cancer free.

Less than two years later we welcomed our second child, Ryan Soto, into our family, a firecracker with a determined personality.

At my baby shower for Ryan, Aunt Susan walked up to me and said, "I found out why your slides were sent to Stanford," she smiled and had a twinkle in her eye. Then she pointed over toward a man with a thick, dark mustache and said, "It was Dr. Greaney. He sent them in." I hadn't seen Dr. Greaney since he gave me the "Battle!" pep talk over fourteen years ago. He was the reason why they caught that it was a more aggressive cancer. He was the reason why I was standing there at my baby shower. I walked up and gave him a big hug. "Dr. Greaney! You're the one who sent my slides to Stanford?" I asked.

"Well, of course I did," he said in his Irish accent with a smile.

"Oh my gosh, I had no idea. Thank you *so much*!" I said while realizing that this simple act was the reason why I was alive and not undertreated for an aggressive cancer. He was the reason why I was able to stand there with my husband and daughter by my side and my son about to be born.

I felt so blessed and grateful to Dr. Greaney and Dr. Siegel for saving my life, and of course to Aunt Susan who had introduced me to them. There were so many people who came together to get me across the finish line. Without each and every one of them I wouldn't have been able to meet my soulmate and have my two wonderful kids.

"Thank you, God, for all of the people who came into my life. They lifted me up and helped me when I needed it the most."

CHAPTER FORTY-ONE

Bless This Broken Road

"You are exactly where you are meant to be." My stepmom would say this to me when things were tough, when I didn't know what direction my life was going in, or what my purpose in life was. It's a phrase that I have heard throughout my life.

It's hard to believe that this is right, but life doesn't always go according to plan. In fact, it seldom does. We encounter things that throw us off course, and the whole time we hope and pray that there is a purpose to it all.

The purpose is our journey. We spend so much of our lives worried about our destination, but it's the journey where you find the beauty in life. It's the small moments you share with others. It's the way a kindness can completely change someone's life. During all of those tough times when I couldn't understand why I wasn't on the right track I was on the right track. I just didn't know it.

Life is full of obstacles. That will never change. What can change is the way you deal with those obstacles. Do you let them stop you, or do you find a way around them to reach your goal? My life has been filled with obstacles that have shaped my journey in a beautiful way. When film school said I couldn't continue with my education, I found a way to continue learning by making a documentary. When my life was not going the way it should after cancer, I devised a plan to escape my situation, which led me to my soulmate. When my dream of introducing Bailey to a dolphin disintegrated, a new dream formed which has affected hundreds of children and their parents. When I was told that I couldn't have kids, I didn't give up, and now I have two.

It's not what happens to you in life that determines your future. It is what you decide to do in those moments of struggle. It is your choices that YOU have control over. You can choose to keep moving and keep finding a path to your dreams and goals.

It all starts with today. It starts with looking at the things you have to be grateful for in your life and, trust me, there is something to be grateful for. It starts with taking a step in that direction towards your goal, even if it is a tiny step. It starts with realizing that every moment we have here is a blessing and not to be taken for granted.

That's how you find your path in life. One day at a time, one step at a time, one getting back up at a time. Your life's journey may have obstacles or times when you seem to go off the path, but ultimately you have control over your choices during all of those times. Choose to be positive, choose to be grateful, choose to get back up, choose not to settle, and choose to find a way. It's the human condition. It's the *Rocky* story that we all want to see. Now, go out and make your own *Rocky* story. I'm rooting for you.

JOY CLAUSEN SOTO

"Bless The Broken Road"
(originally by Nitty Gritty Dirt Band)

I set out on a narrow way many years ago
Hoping I would find true love along the broken road
But I got lost a time or two
Wiped my brow and kept pushing through
I couldn't see how every sign pointed straight to you

Every long lost dream led me to where you are
Others who broke my heart they were like Northern stars
Pointing me on my way into your loving arms
This much I know is true
That God blessed the broken road
That led me straight to you
(Yes He did)

I think about the years I spent just passing through
I'd like to have the time I lost and give it back to you
But you just smile and take my hand
You've been there you understand
It's all part of a grander plan that is coming true

Every long lost dream led me to where you are
Others who broke my heart they were like Northern stars
Pointing me on my way into your loving arms
This much I know is true
That God blessed the broken road
That led me straight to you

Now I'm just rolling home
Into my lover's arms
This much I know is true
That God blessed the broken road
That led me straight to you

That God blessed the broken road
That led me straight to you

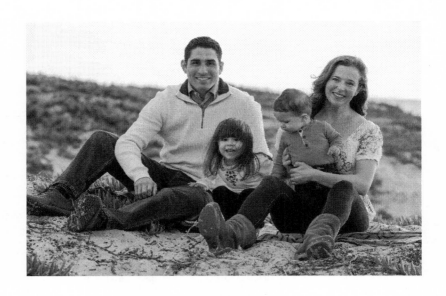

THE END

ACKNOWLEDGMENTS

I t's not just about one person. It's not just about one life. It's about the people along the way who point you in the right direction, who help you when you are down, and who give encouragement when you lose your way. It's the collective whole of your experiences and the people who were there for you whether for a moment or an entire lifetime. I wrote this book, but it took a village of love and encouragement to get here. This is the story of how the book "Joy" came to be.

Back in 2006 I wrote to Zig Ziglar and shared with him how his words had helped me get through cancer. Before I knew it, his company contacted me and offered to fly me to Texas to give a speech to Zig. I'll never forget going into a conference room with his staff seated in front of me, and on the right side in the second row sat Zig Ziglar himself! The same person whose story of being stuck in an airport had helped me turn around a negative situation and start looking at the positives in my life. At the end of the meeting he waited outside for me. He shook my hand and looked into my eyes as he said, "You should write a book, and if you write a book, I'll find you a publisher for it." You would think that would be enough for me to start writing, a proclamation from Zig Ziglar himself, but I didn't start writing. That proclamation came at a point when I was a bit lost in my life. Writing a book didn't feel right at the time.

Five years later after I met my husband and started a program for children with cancer, I went to dinner with Jeni, a co-worker and friend from SeaWorld. She had a ton of questions about my life. I found myself breaking everything down into separate stories, and by the end of our dinner she told me I should write a book. This was the first time that I thought I might actually be able to write something.

Then life gave me another push when our work schedule at SeaWorld started to require late shifts. I didn't have to go into work until 2:30 in the afternoon. Fantastic! I started bringing my computer with me to Starbucks every morning before work. I listened to Adele on repeat as I worked on a chapter. Then I would send that chapter to my stepmom, who would tell me she loved it, hated it, or that it still needed work. Let's be honest. It took a while to get to the "love it" stage, but when I did, it felt *amazing*!

Then there were years that passed by in between when I had my daughter and then my son, when I was just busy living my life. But I still had this book in the background, and I still had people helping me along the way. I remember telling Kristi at work about writing a book and that I needed someone to help me with the grammar. She volunteered her husband, Tyler, who was more than happy to help and meticulously went through it with me. This got me closer to my goal of completing the book and helped me believe that it was worth completing.

In 2017 I hired a professional to give me feedback. He suggested numerous edits. I was so discouraged that part of me wanted to give up at that point, but I kept going until I eventually stopped again.

Then during the pandemic my friend Jeff encouraged me to get on LinkedIn. He taught me how to navigate this platform. If it weren't for him, I wouldn't have started posting, and in turn I wouldn't have posted a goal and deadline to complete my book. This provided the final push to cross the finish line. Plus, I announced it to over 3,000 people. *That* definitely provided a lot of motivation!

Aunt Carol and Ann helped me with the grammar. Aunt Carol took the time to go through it from beginning to end three times and put up with my many grammatical questions. Brigid and Katie gave me additional notes, and Lisa G. improved some of the images in the book.

Then just as I thought I was almost done, I realized I needed to get permission to publish the music lyrics! I was so close! This was another obstacle that got in my way. I took a few days to regroup (okay, I sulked for a few days) and then started working toward securing the music rights. When I found out I had to purchase the copyrights, I decided to remove two of the songs. As I started to rewrite certain chapters, my stepmom decided that the songs were too important to the book. She stepped in and helped me purchase the copyrights. She has always supported me and believed in me.

This book has come together because of the goodness of the people in my life. They listened to me, gave me feedback, encouraged me, and believed that my story was worth sharing with the world. Thank you to everyone who has been a part of this journey.

THANK YOU

-**Alex** for encouraging me during every step of the process. Thank you for always believing in me and supporting my crazy ideas, like writing a book!

-**Christiana** and **Ryan** for loving and supporting me. Thank you for cheering me on along the way. I love you so much!

-**Aunt Susan** for *everything* you did for me. Thank you for introducing me to two incredible doctors and for driving me to my appointments, buying me matzo ball soup, making a ton of food, and welcoming all of my friends into your home. Thank you for holding my hand during the rough times and always being there for me. You are a gift to anyone who knows you.

-**Pacific Mommy Fish** (my stepmom) for listening to me during the good times and the bad times. Thank you for picking me up when I fell down, telling me I was exactly where I was supposed to be, and coming to the rescue when I needed you most. You have been an incredible gift in my life, and I will always be grateful for all of your care, love, and emails telling me to update my Apple IOS software. You are a blessing.

-**Dad** for calling me every single day with words of encouragement and coming out to see me. I love you.

-**Mom** for coming out to help take care of me. You stayed with me in the hospital, made gourmet meals from a microwave, and sneaked Twix bars to me, which I couldn't refuse. Thank you for being there for me.

-**Uncle David** for being a magical uncle. You loved me so much that you found a bear suit at Goodwill for Sean to dress up in and then convinced him to actually wear it! He made me laugh and entertained all of the kids on my floor that day. Magic!

-**Sean** for shaving my head, making me laugh, and dressing up in a bear suit. You know you are loved when someone dresses in a bear suit for you.

-**Melody** for cutting my hair short. It was the stage before I shaved my head. It meant a great deal to have you there. I love you.

-**Dr. Siegel** for being the excellent doctor I needed, for caring about me, and making me feel like a person and not a number. I know you had my best interest at heart, which made me believe in you and the therapy you recommended. I knew I was in the best hands possible for this journey. I will always be beyond grateful to you.

-**Dr. Greaney** for giving me the best, most unexpected motivational speech that belongs in an epic movie and for sending my slides to Stanford. I'm certain I wouldn't be here right now if we hadn't figured out it was a more aggressive cancer.

-**Kevin** for giving up so much to be with me. You were there from week one of finding out I was sick. You coached me through the roughest part of my life and made sure that I crossed that finish line. You were there for every single appointment I had. I know it was a sacrifice for you, and I will forever be grateful and in awe of what you did for me. Words cannot begin to express my eternal gratitude.

-**Brian** for flying out from Boston to see me for two months! I can't believe I am lucky enough to have a friend like you. It was amazing having you by my side. Thank you for helping me walk down that long hallway. I will always cherish that memory.

-**Ann** for giving your time, your love, your energy, and your blood to support me. I'll never forget when you told me that you dreamt of me with gray hair three times. You always told me that if you dreamt about something three times, it would come true. You shared that with me when I was having a rough day and I was scared. You really do know the right thing to say at the right time. Oh, and I have a few gray hairs now!

-**Ryan** for being there for me in the hospital on my first day, last day, and all of those visits in between. Thank you for the warm blue hat I wore religiously after I lost my hair. Thank you for holding my hand during a spinal tap and for the freshly baked cookies you would make and bring to the hospital. You always brought two plates, one for the nurses and one for me.

-**Matt** for hanging out in the hospital with me while I received chemotherapy and for being there whenever I needed you.

-**Karey** for driving up from San Diego to Ventura to see me multiple times. You took my mind off of what was going on and brought a smile to my face. You even drove up to give me a Christmas present, then drove all the way back down to San Diego in one day. You spent six plus hours in the car to simply make sure that I had your present during one of the roughest times in my life. I will always cherish you.

-**Charles** for flying out from Chicago to see me. I told you in the middle of the week that I had cancer, and by the end of the week you were on a plane to be by my side after I had surgery. I'll never forget that.

-**Jim** for making me laugh, as always, helping me eat all of the food Aunt Susan prepared, and staying in your car because you didn't want your dog Mac to come in the house. Thank you for being there for me.

-**Beckie** for spending time with me after my surgery. I remember we all sat around a fire at night laughing and telling stories while roasting marshmallows. I will never forget when you and Karey told me I was your hero over the phone. It brought me to tears then, and it brings me to tears now.

-**Christine** for organizing an army of people to support me and for driving up to keep me company. I always felt your love.

-**Lisa M.** for buying a beautiful blonde wig for me to wear to wear when I lost my hair. I wore it often. Also, thank you for cooking delicious, nutritious food for me when you visited.

-**Art** for accompanying Lisa and also cooking for me.

-**Jerry** for flying out to see me from Chicago. You will always be a great friend.

-**Hoppi** for visiting multiple times both in Ventura and in the hospital. You gave me advice, spent time with me, and let me know that everything I was feeling was "normal."

-**Courtney** for giving blood and spending the night with me in the hospital. It was like a sleepover. You even brought mud masks!

-**Scott** and **Amy** for spending time with me in the hospital. Scott, you inspected my medical notebook and asked me a ton of questions. I could feel your love and how proud you were of me.

-**Mike** and **Kim** for coming to have lunch with me in the hospital. We ate at the McDonalds in the hospital that day. It meant so much to have you there.

-**Mike S.** for giving me DVDs to watch when I was sick. That is when I watched "The Cutting Edge" a sappy love story that was perfect to watch at 2 a.m. when I couldn't sleep.

-**Michelle** for spending time with me in the hospital. We were supposed to have lunch, but instead we had a date in the hospital. Thank you for showing your love.

-**Frank** for complaining about your shoulder hurting after surgery as you took me out to dinner in Ventura. You reminded me that the world didn't revolve around me by talking about your own problems. Plus, you always had such a great attitude. I'm glad we are almost related.

-**Bailey** for being the best roommate and friend I could have asked for at Children's Hospital. You will always live on in my heart and now in this book.

Thank you to everyone who went on this journey with me!